Cardiac Catheterization

Diagnostic Interventions

To my wife, Joyce
My mother and children:
Fredric, Touri and Jeffry

Cardiac Catheterization
Diagnostic Interventions

F. K. NAKHJAVAN, M.D.

Director, Cardiac Catheterization Laboratory,
Albert Einstein Medical Center;
Professor of Medicine,
Temple Medical School
Philadelphia, Pennsylvania

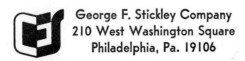
George F. Stickley Company
210 West Washington Square
Philadelphia, Pa. 19106

Contents

Acknowledgments

In the preparation of this book, several physicians have contributed significantly. I thank Dr. R. Paramaswaran, Albert Einstein Medical Center, for his major contribution to the chapter on "Pacing Tachycardia for Detection of Conduction System Abnormalities"; Dr. S. Yazdanfar, Albert Einstein Medical Center, for the collection of hemodynamic and electrophysiological data; and Dr. L. Bentivoglio, Medical College of Pennsylvania, for his suggestions on the exercise chapter. In addition, I greatly appreciate the secretarial work of Mrs. Margaret Kent, and the valuable assistance of Mrs. Grazyna Malz. Finally, I would like to thank Mr. and Mrs. George Stickley for their many excellent ideas for preparation and final touches on this book.

—F. K. NAKHJAVAN, M.D.

Preface

In this book, the diagnostic tests that are commonly used in the cardiac catheterization laboratory and their cardiovascular effects are discussed. The tests are bicycle ergometry, isometric hand grip, atrial pacing, left ventriculography, coronary cineangiography, various maneuvers and pharmacological agents. The aim of the book is to give a general view of these tests since each subject is extensively reported in the literature.

Although stress testing often implies exercise testing, some diagnostic tests such as angiography (volume loading) and pacing tachycardia (increasing the myocardial oxygen demand) cause a stressful effect on the heart. It should be kept in mind that there are technical variations in performing various procedures according to the preference and/or experience of the cardiologist. Certain maneuvers, such as standing or squatting, have significant diagnostic value from a clinical point of view and are not used in the cardiac catheterization laboratory. These are, however, discussed mainly to complement the other related procedures.

—F. K. NAKHJAVAN, M.D.

Foreword

Since Werner Forssmann first catheterized the human heart in 1929, and André Cournand — and Dickinson Richards in the 1940's—demonstrated that heart catheterization was a safe procedure, much has been learned concerning human cardiovascular physiology and clinical heart disease. The application of the technique to the diagnosis of congenital and acquired heart disease is legend.

Cardiac function under a variety of physiological conditions has been extensively studied. These studies have gone far beyond assessing heart function in the resting state.

This book addresses itself to the variety of manipulative procedures employed during cardiac catheterization to further elucidate cardiac function with particular reference to valvular and ischemic heart disease. These procedures include exercise—both dynamic and isometric—atrial pacing, including electrophysiological studies, angiography, various maneuvers and pharmacological agents. These tests are invaluable in the diagnosis, prognosis and in establishing a rational basis for therapy—medical vs. surgical. Furthermore, these tests are of great value in evaluating therapeutic procedures. Although many scientific publications have appeared in the literature, this book brings these procedures, the results, the interpretations and their limitations together in one treatise.

The book will be of value to the internist, cardiologist as well as the student, resident and Fellow in cardiology; all of whom are involved in the total care of the cardiac patient.

HARRY GOLDBERG, M.D.
Professor of Medicine,
Temple Medical School;
Chief of Cardiology Section,
Albert Einstein Medical Center,
Northern Division, Philadelphia.

1
Exercise Testing

In the cardiac catheterization laboratory, exercise testing is generally performed by pedalling a bicycle ergometer in the horizontal position. By using the bicycle ergometer, a fixed amount of work load can be applied for a certain period of time which may vary according to the patient's general condition.

Technical Aspects of Exercise by Bicycle Ergometer

In our cardiac catheterization laboratory, we use a Collins pedal mode ergometer which is fastened to the cardiac catheterization table by an adaptor unit (Fig. I-1). This ergometer provides a work-load which is adjustable over a range of 25–400 watts per second with an accuracy of $\pm 2\%$ of scale. The patient pedals at a speed of more than 35 rpm. Beyond this speed, the work-load remains constant regardless of faster pedalling speed (at 35 rpm, pedal speed reaches the linear portion of the brake unit's hysteresis curve). An appropriate work-load is chosen according to the patient's condition. At this load, the patient pedals for five minutes. It would be desirable to have the patient visit the cardiac catheterization laboratory the day before cardiac catheterization, to be familiarized with the procedure. Since a steady state condition is necessary for accurate measurements of the hemodynamic data during exercise, the following points should be considered:

3

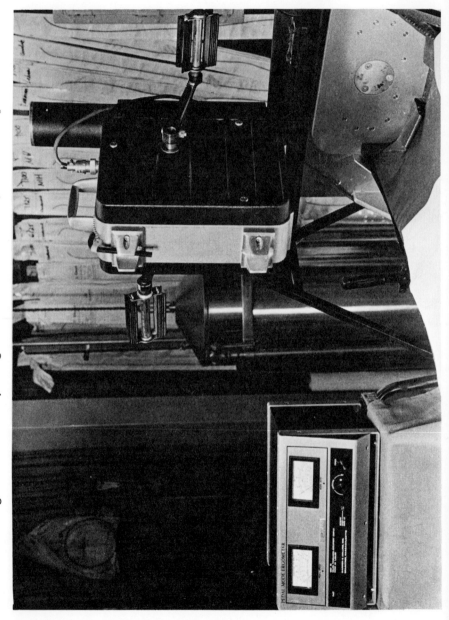

Fig. I-1.   Collins bicycle ergometer in the cardiac catheterization set-up.

Elevating the feet increases the end-diastolic pressures of the ventricles, mainly because of a shift of blood from the legs to the heart; hence control pressure measurements are recorded after the patient's feet are elevated for approximately three minutes on the bicycle ergometer. Hemodynamic measurements are then obtained during the 2nd or 3rd minute of exercise since by this time most of the patients are in a steady state (Fig. I-2).

In our cardiac catheterization laboratory, we perform our studies through the right brachial artery and an antecubital vein. The femoral approach is less suitable for studies during bicycle pedalling. Cardiac output during exercise may be measured by Fick principle, dye dilution or thermodilution techniques. If the Fick principle is used, oxygen consumption and simultaneous systemic arterial and pulmonary arterial blood samples are obtained usually during the 3rd minute of exercise. More simply, cardiac output during the steady state phase of exercise can be obtained by dye dilution or thermodilution techniques. For measurement of pulmonary wedge and pulmonary arterial pressures, the simplest way is to use a balloon-tipped catheter. By inflation of the balloon and subsequent deflation, pulmonary wedge and pulmonary arterial pressures can be readily and rapidly obtained. If an end-hole catheter is used, it should be advanced into the wedge position prior to the exercise testing and subsequently withdrawn to the pulmonary artery on continuous pressure monitoring during the exercise for measurement of pulmonary wedge and arterial pressures and collection of the pulmonary blood sample.

Physiological Response to Exercise

I. Cardiovascular response to exercise: As clearly shown by Braunwald and associates,[1] exercise involves the interaction of: 1) increase in heart rate; 2) changes in stroke volume; 3) in-

6

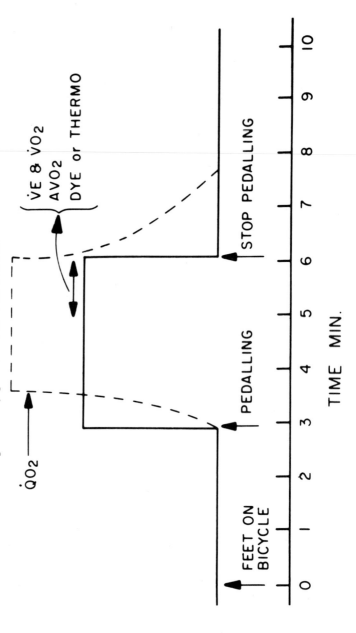

Fig. I-2. Schematic drawing of cardiac output measurement during bicycle pedalling by Fick principle or indicator dilution studies. Control measurements prior to exercise are obtained while the legs are elevated and feet are on the bicycle pedals. A 3-minute period of exercise is usually sufficient. The interrupted line indicates the cardiovascular and pulmonary performance with exercise.

fluence of Frank-Starling mechanism; 4) neurohumoral changes; 5) increase in myocardial contractility. Basically, moderate levels of "supine" exercise cause an increase in heart rate, no significant change in stroke volume (in contrast to exercise in the standing position such as treadmill when stroke volume increases significantly), a decrease in ventricular diastolic volume and an increase in sympathetic tone and myocardial contractility. Because of a decrease in the end-diastolic volume during exercise, it had been thought previously that perhaps the Frank-Starling mechanism is not operative during exercise. However, studies by Ross et al.[2] during pacing tachycardia and also exercise, have clearly demonstrated that ventricular volumes at the same heart rate are larger during exercise than pacing tachycardia. In addition, increased sympathetic activity also contributes to the diminution of ventricular volume during exercise. Generally the increase in heart rate, cardiac output and ventilation during exercise is related to the intensity of the work load. A steady state is usually reached at the end of one minute of exercise, and hence cardiac output should be measured after the first minute of exercise. However, in patients with severe depression of myocardial function, it may take longer to reach the steady state or they may actually never reach this point.

Since cardiac output is the product of

$$\frac{\text{oxygen consumption}}{\text{systemic } AV_{O_2} \text{ difference}}$$

an insufficient increase of cardiac output during exercise may be related to the inadequate increase of oxygen consumption and/or excessive increase in the systemic arteriovenous oxygen difference. The increase in cardiac output in relation to oxygen uptake in normal subjects is shown in Figure I-3. For each 600 ml increase in cardiac output, there is 100 cm³ increase in oxygen consump-

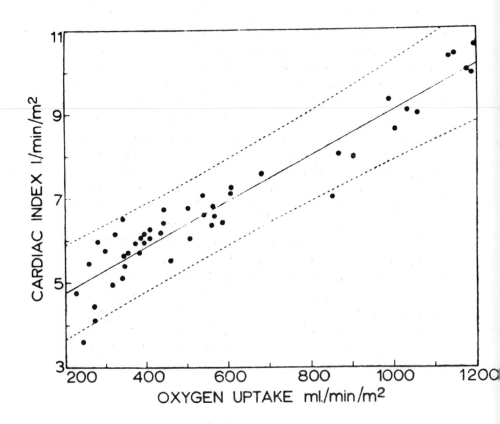

Fig. I-3. The relationship between cardiac index and oxygen uptake during exercise in the supine position in normal subjects. Regression line and 95% confidence limits are shown. (From Donald et al. The effect of exercise on the cardiac output and circulatory dynamics of normal subjects. Clin. Sci. 14:37, 1955.)

tion. During exercise, there is also an increase in systemic AV_{O_2} difference. The relationship between AV_{O_2} difference and O_2 uptake is shown in Figure I-4.

After cessation of exercise, cardiac output returns to the control value in approximately two minutes. Often the return of cardiac output to the pre-exercise level is not measured in the cardiac catheterization laboratory. However, if the exercise has to be repeated, 20–30 minutes should be allowed until the next exercise test for complete return of the cardiovascular and ventilatory changes to the control state.

Note: Since cardiac output is also the product of stroke volume X heart rate, an increase in cardiac output may be the result of an increase in either a stroke volume or heart rate. Although controversy in regard to the increase in stroke volume during exercise has existed for a long time, as was mentioned previously, it is now generally agreed that during supine exercise the changes in stroke volume are not marked, i.e., stroke volume may not change, decrease or increase slightly. Hence tachycardia of exercise is the dominant factor in increasing the cardiac output during submaximal supine exercise. It should also be mentioned that during exercise in the upright position, stroke volume does increase. However, cardiac output and stroke volume at rest in the upright position are both lower than in the supine position.

Intracardiac pressures during exercise: Although it had been thought previously that pulmonary arterial pressure does not increase significantly during moderate degrees of exercise, subsequent studies have shown that with moderate levels of exercise, when the cardiac output increases two to three times, there is also a moderate increase in pulmonary arterial pressure.[3] The pressure in the pulmonary artery is dependent on several factors which include: pulmonary flow (i.e., cardiac output), left atrial pressure, pulmonary venous pressure, pulmonary vascular resistance

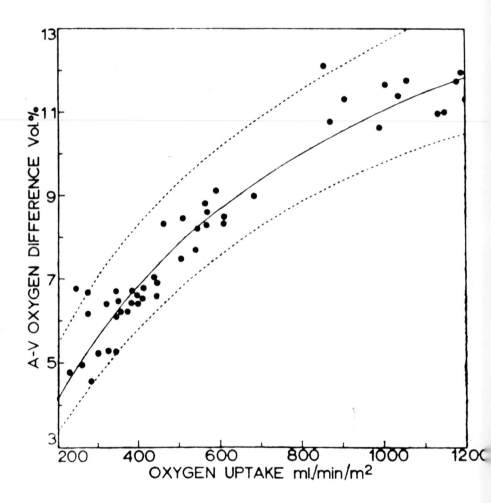

Fig. I-4. The relationship between arteriovenous oxygen difference and oxygen uptake during supine exercise. (From Donald et al. The effect of exercise on the cardiac output and circulatory dynamics of normal subjects. Clin. Sci. 14:37, 1955.

and also intrathoracic pressure. The left atrial pressure itself is subject to the flow, left atrial compliance, mitral valve resistance and the compliance and function of the left ventricle. It is now known that the pulmonary arterial pressure and pulmonary wedge pressure (Fig. I-5) increase during exercise. However, since the increase in flow during exercise is more than the increase in pulmonary arterial pressure, there is an actual diminution in pulmonary vascular resistance. In older subjects, the increase in pulmonary wedge and pulmonary arterial pressures are higher than in younger ones.[4] Similarly, during exercise there is an increase in the systemic systolic, diastolic and mean blood pressures; however, because of a significant increase in cardiac output, the systemic vascular resistance is decreased.

Evaluation of the cardiovascular response to supine exercise: Measurement of left ventricular end-diastolic pressure (LVEDP) and its relationship to stroke volume or stroke work index (SWI) is of particular importance in differentiating between patients with normal and abnormal cardiac response to exercise. In patients with a normal left ventricular response, there is no significant change in LVEDP (not exceeding 12 mmHg) while SWI increases. On the other hand, in patients with abnormal left ventricular function, LVEDP increases.[5] In some of these patients, SWI increases, while in others it may even diminish (Fig. I-6). In addition, in patients with depressed myocardial function, the relationship between oxygen consumption and cardiac output or AVO_2 difference usually shows a diminished cardiac output and a wide AVO_2 difference for a given $\dot{V}O_2$ (exercise factor < 600 ml/min. increase in cardiac output for each 100 ml $\dot{V}O_2$/min.). The diminished response of cardiac output to exercise may be because of myocardial failure, increased resistance to flow (i.e., pulmonary hypertension, mitral stenosis, aortic stenosis, etc.), regurgitant lesions and dyskinetic areas of the heart, etc. Hence, interpretation of an abnormal myocardial

12

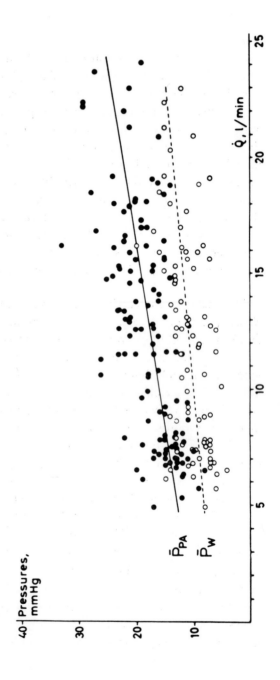

Fig. I-5. The relationship between pulmonary arterial mean pressure (P̄PA), pulmonary wedge pressure (P̄W) and cardiac output (Q̇.L/min) during rest and supine exercise in healthy young men and women. Solid symbols indicate men; open symbols indicate women. (From Ekelund and Holmgren. Circ. Res. 20 (Suppl. I): 1–33, 1967.)

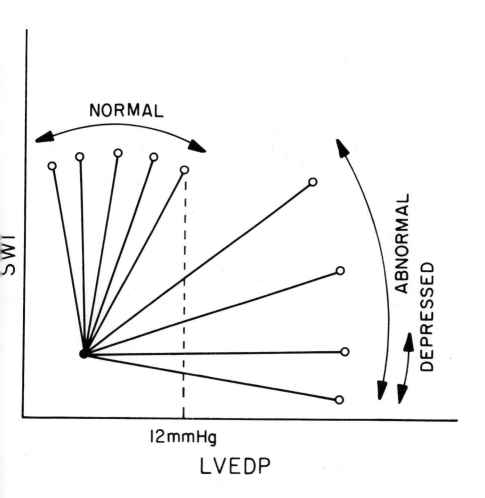

Fig. I-6. Relationship between left ventricular end-diastolic pressure (LVEDP) and stroke work index (SWI). (Modified from Ross, J., Jr., et al. Left ventricular performance during muscular exercise in patients with and without cardiac dysfunction. Circulation 34:597, 1966.)

response to exercise should be done with caution and in light of the underlying cardiac condition. In this regard, assessment of myocardial contractility using various angiographic, radio-isotopic, echocardiographic and force velocity measurements would be of particular importance.

II. Ventilatory response to exercise: It is well known that exercise is the most important factor in increasing the ventilation. The observations of Krogh and Lindhard[6] and subsequently Asmussen and Nielsen[7] have shown that the ventilation increases actually before the onset of exercise, and this is unrelated to the level of work that the subject will subsequently perform. This initial increase in ventilation is most likely caused by neuro-humoral influences.

Since ventilation and oxygen consumption during exercise are linearly related to the intensity of work load, a simple relationship between ventilation and oxygen consumption exists for sub-maximal levels of oxygen consumption, i.e., up to levels of oxygen consumption of 2 1/min. The slope of the line, i.e.,

$$\frac{VE\ (BTPS)}{\dot{V}O_2\ (STPD)} = 22\text{--}25$$

in normal subjects. At higher levels of work, the increase in ventilation is somewhat greater in relation to oxygen consumption. With myocardial dysfunction, an inappropriate response of ventilation in relation to oxygen consumption may occur.

III. Myocardial metabolic response during exercise: Myocardium uses as its most important substrates, fatty acids, glucose, lactate and to a smaller degree, pyruvate. Other substances, such as ketones and amino acids, are used to a much lesser degree.

Myocardial extraction is usually proportionate to the substrate concentration of the arterial blood and normally fatty acids are utilized more than carbohydrates. Since myocardial oxygen extraction is quite high (70%) in the resting state, the increase in myocardial oxygen consumption is mainly met by a rise in coronary blood flow. However, in patients with coronary artery disease, the increase in coronary flow is not adequate for the increase in myocardial demand. Normally, myocardium relies on aerobic metabolism. Figure I-7 demonstrates the normal myocardial metabolic pathway. Fatty acid is mostly converted to acetyl coenzyme A. Lactate is extracted by the myocardium from the blood and converted to pyruvate. Pyruvic acid is rapidly decarboxylated to form acetyl CoA (and hence is not converted to lactic acid) and thus myocardium does not normally produce lactic acid. The following formula shows the reaction between pyruvic acid and lactic acid: pyruvic acid + NADH + H$^+$ ⇌ lactic acid + NAD$^+$. Pyruvic acid will accumulate if there is increased glycolytic production of pyruvic acid or decreased utilization of pyruvic acid by Kreb's cycle, both of which occur during hypoxia. Accumulation and increase of pyruvic acid will shift the above reaction toward lactic acid production.

Figure I-8 shows the myocardial metabolic pathway during hypoxia. The anaerobic metabolism, however, is not adequate to maintain the myocardial energy demands for a sustained period of time. The high energy phosphates during ischemia diminish rapidly and myocardial contractility becomes depressed. During steady state resting condition, myocardium extracts lactic acid (10% or more).[8] Diminution of coronary blood flow by 25 per cent of the control when coronary sinus PO$_2$ is less than 10 mmHg usually results in lactate production.[9]

Abnormalities of myocardial metabolism are generally described in the following terms:

1. *Myocardial lactate production:* As was mentioned previously, myocardium normally extracts lactate and lactate production is generally due to an increased glycolysis or decreased utilization of pyruvate by Kreb's cycle, either of which occurs with hypoxia.

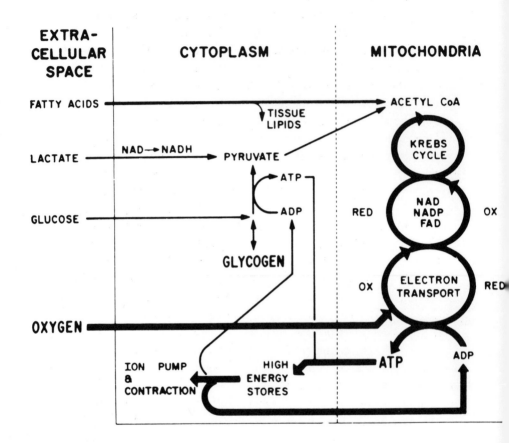

Fig. I-7. Energy pathway in the normal myocardium. (From Scheuer. Myocardial metabolism in cardiac hypoxia. Am. J. Cardiol. 19:385, 1967.)

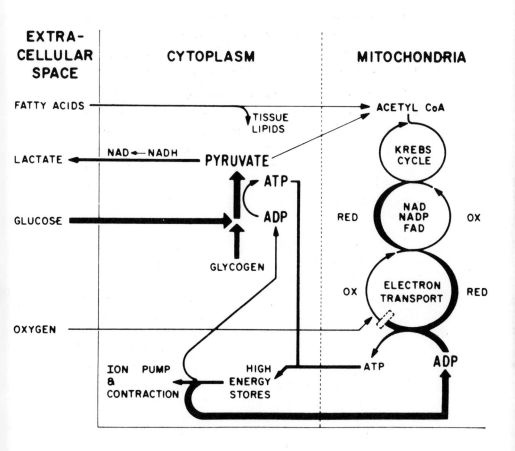

Fig. I-8. Energy pathway in the hypoxic myocardium. (From Scheuer. Myocardial metabolism in cardiac hypoxia. Am. J. Cardiol. 19:385, 1967.)

2. Diminished lactate extraction: As was mentioned previously, myocardium extracts more than 10 per cent of the arterial lactate. Thus, diminished lactate extraction is considered to be an indication of myocardial hypoxia.

3. Coronary sinus lactate-pyruvate ratio (L/P$_{cs}$): Studies by Neill[10] have shown that more than a 10 per cent change in L/P$_{cs}$ with no significant change in arterial lactate-pyruvate ratio (less than 7%) during coronary artery stress (such as pacing tachycardia) is an indication of myocardial hypoxia. In our experience, during exercise the L/P ratio changes more than 7 per cent and hence this parameter is not useful.

4. Excess lactate: The concept of excess lactate as introduced by Huckabee[11,12] is the amount of lactate which is produced in excess of that produced by the increase in pyruvate. The formula for calculation of excess lactate is: $XL = (L_{cs} - L_{art}) - (P_{cs} - P_{art}) (L_{art}/P_{art})$. Since pyruvate concentration is quite small and pyruvate is subject to spontaneous decarboxylation, and also because of theoretical problems with the use of the excess lactate concept as an indicator of myocardial hypoxia, lactate production or decreased extraction are more often used.

Myocardial metabolic studies during exercise are often employed in patients with chest pain (syndrome X) or coronary artery disease. It is of interest that although physical exertion is the most common cause of angina in patients with coronary artery disease, the metabolic studies during exercise often do not correlate closely with patients' symptomatology or electrocardiographic abnormalities.[13] Thus, during exercise–induced angina, there is often an ischemic ST pattern on the electrocardiogram, elevated LVEDP, depression of myocardial contractility or function while myocardial lactate metabolism is often normal. This may be due to the rising level of arterial lactate during exercise and may not represent the true metabolic state of the heart.[14]

Another possibility is the redistribution of coronary blood flow: although there are areas in the myocardium which are ischemic and produce lactate, they are outweighed by the normal areas and so the integrated effect of coronary sinus sampling results in a positive myocardial arteriovenous lactate difference. Studies by Herman et al.[15] on zonal myocardial ischemia have shown that by sampling at various sites of the coronary sinus, the ischemic area of the myocardium may be selectively localized. On the other hand, measurement of coronary blood flow and myocardial oxygen extraction during resting control state, supine exercise and isoproterenol infusion (1–5 μg/min) has not differentiated patients with coronary artery disease from normal subjects.[8]

Note: Among the three types of myocardial stress tests which are often used, i.e., exercise, pacing tachycardia and isoproterenol infusion, pacing tachycardia has the greatest yield as far as myocardial lactate metabolism is concerned. Isoproterenol is not used often since it promotes glycolysis and lactate production irrespective of myocardial ischemia.[16]

Exercise Testing In Heart Disease

Mitral Stenosis: Exercise causes an increase in mitral valve gradient and left atrial pressure reflected in the pulmonary circulation. This increase is due to the rise in cardiac output and heart rate, either of which increases the mitral valve gradient and left atrial pressure independently. Since, as was mentioned previously, the effects of exercise are partly due to the integrated influence of tachycardia and catecholamine stimulation, we studied the influence of these two in a group of patients with mitral stenosis and normal sinus rhythm. Figure I-9 shows simultaneous left ventricular and left atrial pressures in a patient with mitral stenosis during control state, supine exercise, isoproterenol infusion and tachycardia by right atrial pacing. The latter two were performed at the same rate as that achieved during exercise. The left atrial pressure and left ventricular-left atrial diastolic pressure gradients are highest during exercise.[17] Figure I-10 shows the changes in di-

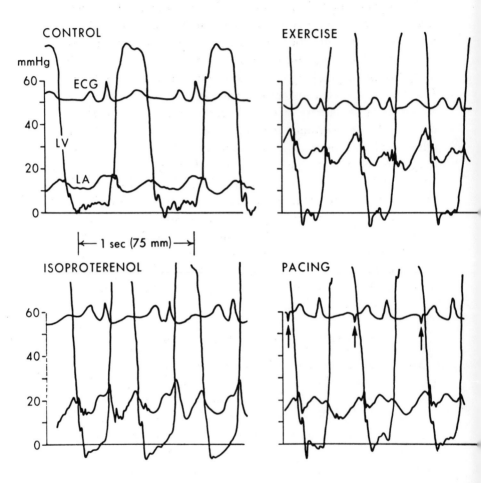

Fig. I-9. Simultaneous pressure recording of left ventricle (LV) and left atriu (LA) during control state, exercise, isoproterenol infusion and pacing in a repr sentative study. (From Nakhjavan et al. Hemodynamic effects of exercise, cat cholamine stimulation and tachycardia in mitral stenosis and sinus rhythm at con parable heart rates. Am. J. Cardiol. 23:659, 1969.)

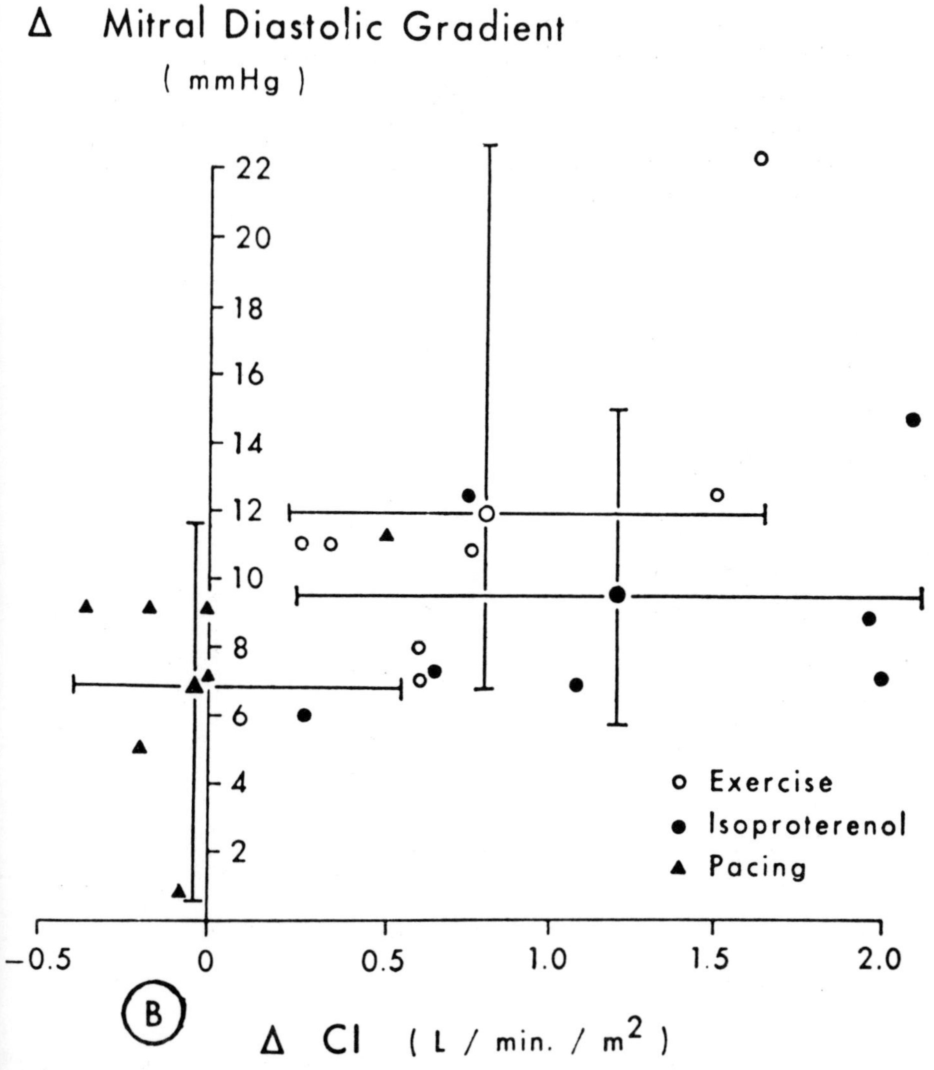

Δ Mitral Diastolic Gradient
(mmHg)

Fig. I-10.   Relationship between changes in mitral diastolic gradient and cardiac index. The effects of exercise are similar to those of infusion of isoproterenol. (From Nakhjavan et al. Hemodynamic effects of exercise, catecholamine stimulation and tachycardia in mitral stenosis and sinus rhythm at comparable heart rates. Am. J. Cardiol. 23:659, 1969.)

22

astolic mitral valve gradient as related to changes in cardiac index. It should be noted that pacing tachycardia increases the mitral valve diastolic gradient but does not change the cardiac output significantly. When exercise studies were performed after beta-blockade with propranolol, heart rate, cardiac output and mitral valve gradient diminished.[18] When the heart rate is kept constant at the same rate as during the control supine exercise by right

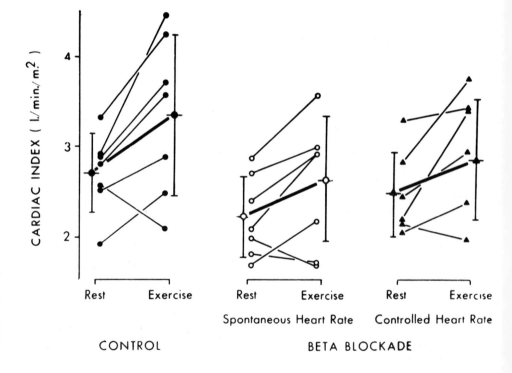

Fig. I-11. Cardiac index (1/min/m²) during control state (rest and exercise) and after Beta blockade during spontaneous and controlled heart rates. Mean ± SD are shown by horizontal bars. (From Nakhjavan et al. Analysis of influence of catecholamine and tachycardia during supine exercise in patients with mitral stenosis and sinus rhythm. Br. Heart J. 31:753, 1969.)

atrial pacing, the mitral valve gradient increases to the same level as the control exercise with spontaneous heart rate, while cardiac output remains lower than the control state (Figs. I-11 and I-12).

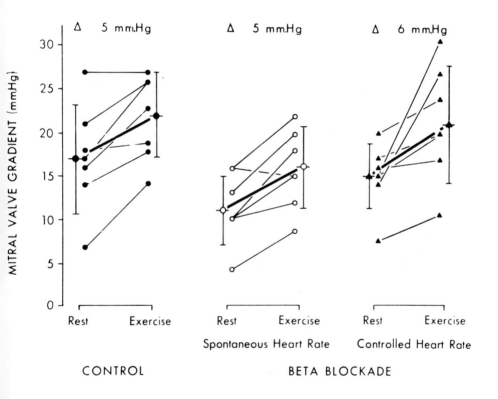

Fig. I-12. Mitral valve diastolic pressure gradient at control state and after Beta blockade during spontaneous and controlled heart rate. Mean ± SD are shown by horizontal bars. (From Nakhjavan et al. Analysis of influence of catecholamine and tachycardia during supine exercise in patients with mitral stenosis and sinus rhythm. Br. Heart J. 31:753, 1969.)

Mitral Regurgitation: Hemodynamic studies during exercise in patients with mitral regurgitation are similar to mitral stenosis except for pulmonary wedge pressure and left ventricular volume. Studies by Draper and associates[19] have shown that during exercise, patients with mitral regurgitation have a lesser increase (or actually a decrease) in cardiac output compared to patients with mitral stenosis, since in the former there is a marked widening of systemic arteriovenous oxygen difference.

Aortic Valvular Disease: The response of the cardiovascular system during exercise in aortic stenosis is usually abnormal in that the increase in cardiac output is generally less than would be expected and is similar to patients with aortic regurgitation. This is shown by Goldberg et al.[20] in their original studies (Figs. I-13 and I-14). Similar studies have been reported by Gorlin et al.[21] Anderson and co-workers[22] studied 32 patients with aortic stenosis, 18 of whom had minimal or no aortic regurgitation. The average cardiac index at rest was 2.5 l/min/m² and increased to 3.8 l/min/m² during exercise. Of particular interest was the fact that during exercise the mean systolic pressure across the aortic valve decreased or remained unchanged in 11 patients. The left ventricular and aortic systolic and diastolic pressures increased.

Analysis of the left ventricular stroke work index as related to left ventricular end-diastolic pressure differentiated the patients with well-functioning ventricles from those with poor myocardial function. In the former, there was an average increase of 39 per cent in stroke work index (SWI) associated with a 69 per cent

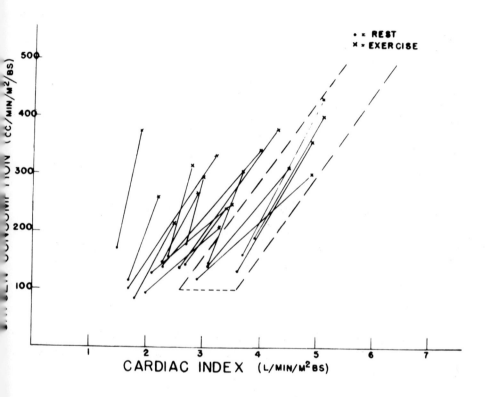

Fig. I-13. The relationship of the oxygen consumption and the cardiac index at ~st and during exercise in 18 patients with aortic stenosis. The area enclosed by the ~oken lines represents the normal values at rest and during exercise as determined ~ normal individuals. (From Goldberg et al. The dynamics of aortic valvular ~sease. Am. Heart J. 47:527, 1954.)

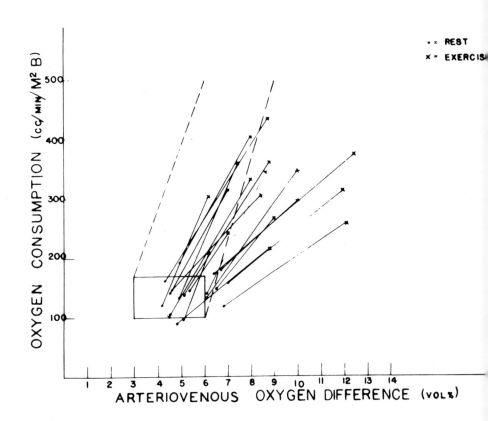

Fig. I-14.   The relationship of the oxygen consumption and arteriovenous oxyg difference at rest and during exercise in 18 patients with aortic stenosis. The ar enclosed by the rectangle and the straight lines extended from its extremities rep sent the range of normal values. (From Goldberg et al. The dynamics of aor valvular disease. Am. Heart J. 47:527, 1954.)

increase in LVEDP. In the latter group, SWI increased 1.3 per cent, while LVEDP increased by 129 per cent. It should be mentioned that in patients with aortic stenosis, the atrial contribution to the cardiac output is of particular importance. As shown by Stott et al.,[23] in aortic stenosis the atrial contribution to cardiac output is greater than in normal subjects (39% in aortic stenosis vs. 26% in the control group).

Coronary Artery Disease: Studies during exercise in patients with coronary artery disease have shown that the cardiac hemodynamic response in such patients is often abnormal. Studies by McCallister and associates[24] have shown that the left ventricular end-diastolic pressure during exercise rose to 30 ± 8 mmHg in 19 patients with coronary artery disease. There was no statistically significant difference in patients who developed angina during the exercise testing compared to those who did not develop angina. The rise in LVEDP in patients with coronary artery disease may be partly related to the extent of disease as shown by Saltups et al.[25] Wiener and co-workers[26] have shown that the rise in LVEDP occurs prior to the onset of angina or electrocardiographic evidence of ischemia. McCallister and colleagues[24] have shown abnormality of myocardial performance in 68 per cent (13/19) of the patients with coronary artery disease, i.e., a significant rise in the left ventricular end-diastolic pressure without a significant increase in left ventricular stroke index. The marked increase in LVEDP in patients with coronary artery disease may be related to diminished myocardial compliance and hence the relationship between LVEDP and LVSWI should be interpreted with caution.

Thus, without knowing the left ventricular volume and the possible development of mitral regurgitation or ventricular dyskinesia secondary to papillary muscle dysfunction during exercise —with resultant diminution in cardiac output in the face of a depressed ventricular function curve—one may not speak unequivocally of "myocardial" failure. Indeed, changes in diastolic pressure-volume relationship of the heart are demonstrated during pacing induced angina.[27]

References

1. Braunwald, E., Sonnenblick, E. H., Ross, J., Jr., Glick, G. and Epstein, S. E. An analysis of the cardiac response to exercise. Circ. Res. 20 (Supplement I):1–44, 1967.
2. Ross, J., Jr., Linhart, J. W. and Braunwald, E. Effects of changing heart rate in man by electrical stimulation of the right atrium: Studies at rest, during exercise and with isoproterenol. Circulation 32:549, 1965.
3. Fowler, N. O. (Editorial) The normal pulmonary arterial pressure-flow relationship during exercise. Am. J. Med. 47:1, 1969.
4. Ekelund, L. G. and Holmgren, A. Central hemodynamics during exercise. Circ. Res. 20 (Supplement I):1–33, 1967.
5. Ross, J., Jr., Gault, J. H., Mason, D. T., Linhart, J. W. and Braunwald, E. Left ventricular performance during muscular exercise in patients with and without cardiac dysfunction. Circulation 34:597, 1966.
6. Krogh, A. and Lindhard, J. The regulation of respiration and circulation during the initial stages of muscular work. J. Physiol. 47:112, 1913.
7. Asmussen, E. and Nielsen, M. Studies on the initial changes in respiration at the transition from rest to work and from work to rest. Acta Physiol. Scand. 16:270, 1948.
8. Cohen, L. S., Elliott, W. C., Klein, M. D. and Gorlin, R. Coronary heart disease: Clinical, cinearteriographic and metabolic correlations. Am. J. Cardiol. 17:153, 1966.

9. Shea, T. M., Watson, R. M., Piotrowski, S. F., Dermksian, G. and Case, R. B. Anaerobic myocardial metabolism. Am. J. Physiol. 203:463, 1962.
10. Neill, W. A. Myocardial hypoxia and anaerobic metabolism in coronary heart disease. Am. J. Cardiol. 22:507, 1968.
11. Huckabee, W. E. Relationships of pyruvate and lactate during anaerobic metabolism. II. Exercise and formation of O_2 debt. J. Clin. Invest. 37:255, 1958.
12. Huckabee, W. E. Abnormal resting blood lactate. I. The significance of hyperlactatemia in hospitalized patients. Am. J. Med. 30:833, 1961.
13. Parker, J. O., West, R. O., Care, R. B. and Chiong, M. A. Temporal relationships of myocardial lactate metabolism, left ventricular function and S-T segment depression during angina precipitated by exercise. Circulation 40:97, 1969.
14. Zierler, K. L. Theory of the use of arteriovenous concentration differences for measuring metabolism in steady and non-steady states. J. Clin. Invest. 40:2111, 1961.
15. Herman, M., Elliott, W. C. and Gorlin, R. An electrocardiographic, anatomic, and metabolic study of zonal myocardial ischemia in coronary heart disease. Circulation 35:834, 1967.
16. Winterscheid, L. C., Bruce, R. A., Blumberg, J. B. and Merendino, K. A. Carbohydrate metabolism of isolated canine heart. Circ. Res. 12:76, 1963.
17. Nakhjavan, F. K., Katz, M. R., Shedrovilsky, H., Maranhao, V. and Goldberg, H. Hemodynamic effects of exercise, catecholamine stimulation and tachycardia in mitral stenosis and sinus rhythm at comparable heart rates. Am. J. Card. 23:659, 1969.
18. Nakhjavan, F. K., Katz, M. R., Maranhao, V. and Goldberg, H. Analysis of influence of catecholamine and tachycardia during supine exercise in patients with mitral stenosis and sinus rhythm. Br. Heart J. 31:753, 1969.
19. Draper, A., Heimbecker, R., Daley, R., Carrol, D., Mudd, G., Wells, R., Falholt, W., Andrus, E. C. and Bing, R. J. Physiologic studies in mitral valvular disease. Circulation 3:531, 1951.
20. Goldberg, H., Bakst, A. A. and Bailey, C. P. The dynamics of aortic valvular disease. Am. Heart J. 47:527, 1954.
21. Gorlin, R., McMillan, I. K. R., Medd, W. E., Matthews, M. B. and Daley, R. Dynamics of the circulation in aortic valvular disease. Am. J. Med. 18:855, 1955.

22. Anderson, F. L., Tsagaris, T. J., Tikoff, G., Torne, J., Schmidt, A. M. and Kuida, H. Hemodynamic effects of exercise in patients with aortic stenosis. Am. J. Med. 46:872, 1969.
23. Stott, D. K., Marpole, D. C. F., Bristow, J. D., Kloster, F. E. and Griswold, H. E. The role of left atrial transport in aortic and mitral stenosis. Circulation 41:1031, 1970.
24. McCallister, B. D., Yipintsoi, T., Hallerman, F. J., Wallace, R. B. and Frye, R. L. Left ventricular performance during mild supine leg exercise in coronary artery disease. Circulation 37: 922, 1968.
25. Saltups, A., McCallister, B. D., Hallerman, F. J., Wallace, R. B., Smith, R. E. and Frye, R. L. Left ventricular hemodynamics in patients with coronary artery disease and in normal subjects. Am. J. Med. 50:8, 1971.
26. Wiener, L., Dwyer, E. M., Jr., and Case, J. W. Left ventricular hemodynamics in exercise induced angina pectoris. Circulation 38:240, 1968.
27. Barry, W. H., Brooker, J. Z., Alderman, E. L. and Harrison, D. C. Changes in diastolic stiffness and tone of the left ventricle during angina pectoris. Circulation 49:255, 1974.

2

Isometric Exercise

Isometric exercise test (static exercise as compared to dynamic exercise) is a commonly used stress test to elicit myocardial abnormalities. It may be used clinically at the bedside or in the cardiac catheterization laboratory. Clinically, it is easily done by asking the patient to make a fist for about a minute, while in the laboratory a dynamometer is used and the amount of developed tension by a muscle group (generally the forearm muscles) is graded. This is usually done between 15 to 35 per cent of maximal voluntary contraction (MVC). In our cardiac catheterization laboratory, we have been using a dynamometer* (Fig. II-1) at 30 per cent of MVC using the left hand (since cardiac catheterization studies are performed from the right arm in most cases). Others have used a balloon dynamometer.[1]

Physiological response to isometric exercise: The physiological response to isometric exercise is mainly related to the relative tension of the muscle group and not the muscle bulk, i.e., the response is not additive.[2] It is initiated by a strong reflex (originating in the muscles), which causes a major involvement by the cardiovascular system. There are basically three changes:

---

* Stolting Co., Chicago 24, Ill., U.S.A.

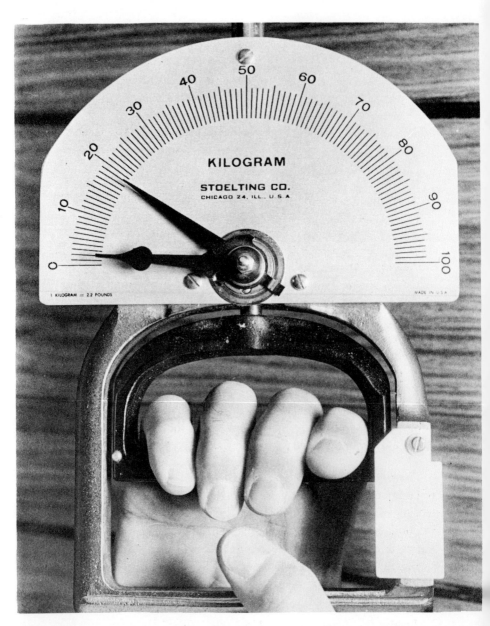

Fig. II-1. The dynamometer which is currently used in our cardiac catheterization laboratory.

1. An increase in heart rate.
2. An increase in cardiac output secondary to an increase in heart rate with no significant change in stroke volume.
3. A significant increase in systemic blood pressure secondary to an increase in cardiac output with no significant change in systemic vascular resistance.

If the first response (tachycardia) is inadequate, then the stroke volume or systemic vascular resistance may increase. Also, in elderly patients, systemic vascular resistance may increase. The above changes return to control levels shortly after cessation of the isometric exercise. It should be mentioned that the isometric exercise can induce its characteristic pressure response and tachycardia even during dynamic exercise.

Isometric exercise to determine left ventricular performance: The hand grip test has been used to differentiate patients with abnormal myocardial function by relating the changes in the left ventricular end-diastolic pressure (LVEDP) to stroke work. Figure II-2 shows schematically the normal and abnormal response to isometric hand grip. The effects of isometric hand grip on the left ventricular pressure in a patient with coronary artery disease is shown in Figure II-3. In a study reported by Helfant, De Villa and Meister,[3] LVEDP increased by 9.7 mmHg ± 1.7 (SEM) in patients with depressed myocardial function and 2.1 mmHg ± 0.7 (SEM) in the control group. Ventricular function curves relating LVEDP to the stroke work index before and after hand grip were steep in normal subjects and flat or less steep in patients with myocardial dysfunction.[3,4]

Isometric exercise test at the bedside: Because of the profound physiological effects of the isometric exercise test and its ease of performance, it is used frequently at the bedside to detect abnormal myocardial function or to differentiate certain murmurs.

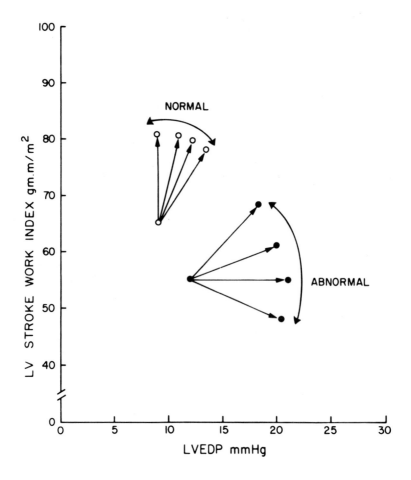

Fig. II-2. Schematic demonstration of the effects of isometric hand grip in normal and abnormal hearts. In normal hearts the increase in left ventricular stroke work index is significant, while there is only a moderate rise in LVEDP. In contrast, in abnormal hearts the increase in LVEDP is much more marked.

At the bedside, it is usually performed by asking the patient to make a firm fist while the examiner listens to the heart. The degree of pressure effect may be determined by measuring the blood pressure. Precordial bulges indicative of asynchrony of contraction or atrial "kicks"—S_4 and S_3—may appear or become more marked. The murmurs of aortic stenosis or idiopathic subaortic stenosis diminish while the murmur of mitral regurgitation increases. (See Chapter VI for details.)

Isometric exercise test and myocardial metabolic studies: Since various stress tests, particularly pacing tachycardia, are often used for their effect on myocardial metabolism, isometric exercise has also been used for such studies. In our laboratory, we have used the hand grip test as a stress test for myocardial metabolic studies.[5] Compared to pacing tachycardia, the hand grip test is not as sensitive for detecting myocardial ischemia as is evidenced by myocardial lactate abnormalities (Fig. II-4). Even when hand grip was combined with pacing tachycardia (which caused the highest tension time index as a determinant of myocardial oxygen consumption), myocardial lactate abnormalities were more frequent during pacing tachycardia. The rising level of arterial blood lactate probably causes a positive myocardial arteriovenous lactate difference even though myocardial ischemia may be present. Similar results are seen with dynamic exercise. Relevant hemodynamic data in 25 patients who had myocardial metabolic studies performed in our laboratory are shown in Table II-1.[5]

Comparison between dynamic and static exercise: The cardiovascular response to dynamic vs. static exercise has several important differences.[6] These are schematically shown below:

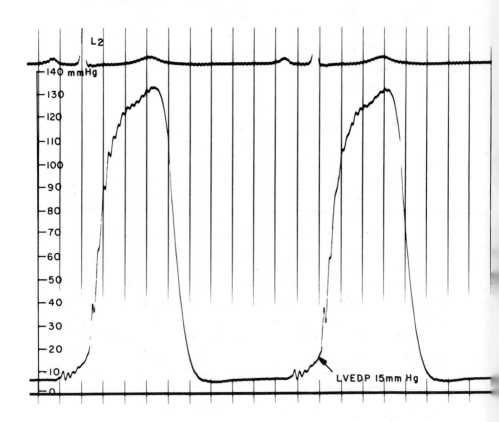

Fig. II-3A. Isometric hand grip (at 30% of MVC) in a patient with coronary
artery disease. Control.

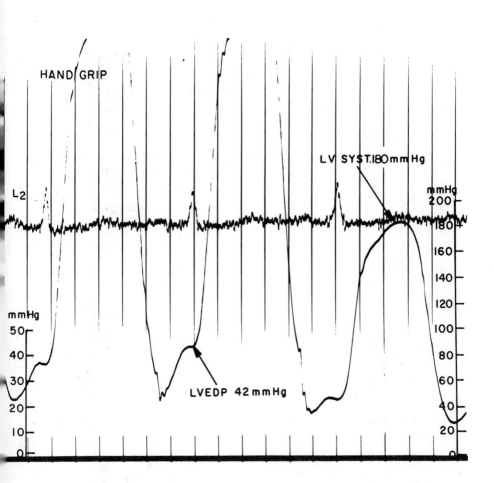

Fig. II-3B. Hand grip: note the marked rise in LVEDP. Left ventricular stroke work index decreased from a control of 59 gm M/m² to 45.5 gm M/m².

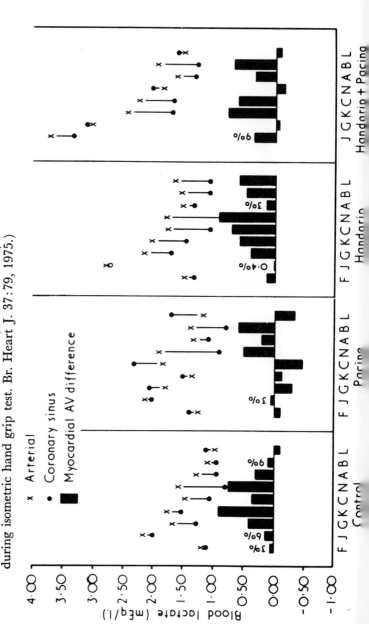

Fig. II-4. Myocardial metabolic studies in nine patients with chest pain and myocardial lactate abnormalities. Arterial, coronary sinus and myocardial arteriovenous lactate difference during control state, pacing tachycardia, hand grip and combined hand grip plus pacing tachycardia are shown. Percentage figures denote the myocardial lactate extraction as a percentage of arterial content. Hand grip and hand grip plus pacing tachycardia does not cause myocardial lactate abnormalities as often as pacing tachycardia. (From Nakhjavan, et al. Myocardial lactate metabolism during isometric hand grip test. Br. Heart J. 37:79, 1975.)

	Heart Rate	Systemic Pressure			Cardiac Output	Systemic Vascular Resistance
		Syst.	Diast.	Mean		
Dynamic Exercise	↑ + + + +	↑ + +	↑ + or ↔	or + + to + +	↑ + + + +	↓ + + + +
Isometric Hand Grip	↑ + +	↑ + + + +	↑ + + + +	↑ + + + +	↑ + +	↔ or ↑ (elderly)

Studies by Lindquist, Spangler and Blount[7] have shown that during isometric hand grip compared to dynamic exercise at comparable heart rates, there was no change in pre-ejection period and isovolumic contraction time, while QS_2 and left ventricular ejection time shortened. In addition, the triple product (HR × left ventricular ejection time × systolic BP) as an estimate of myocardial O_2 consumption was higher during the isometric hand grip test. Because of a marked increase in blood pressure and a moderate increase in cardiac output, isometric exercise is poorly tolerated by patients with compromised myocardial function.

Isometric hand grip test as a stress test during left ventriculography: Since patients with coronary artery disease may develop abnormalities of myocardial contractions during a stress test (such as pacing tachycardia), left ventriculography has been used during the hand grip test in conjunction with atrial pacing.[8] It was shown that the combination of atrial pacing and isometric hand grip may identify segmental abnormalities of the left ventricular contractions in patients with coronary artery disease. Also, studies by Flessas et al.[9] relating the left ventricular end-diastolic pressure to left ventricular volumes have shown that in patients with coronary artery disease during isometric exercise,

TABLE II-1.   Hemodynamic studies in 25 patients who had myocardial metabolic Normal lactate (16 patients). From Nakhjavan et al, MYOCARDIAL LACTATE Journal 37:79, 1975.

		Age (yr)	Heart rate/ min	S	Aortic pressure (mmHg) D	M
Group I: abnormal lactate						
Control	Mean	49.6	74	142	76	102
	±SE	2.4	4.4	9.2	3.2	5.8
Pacing	Mean		132	140	90	108
	±SE		4.0	7.5	2.2	4.6
Hand grip	Mean		90	167	97	125
	±SE		5.5	7.2	4.2	4.5
Pacing plus	Mean		133	169	109	131
hand grip	±SE		5.0	9.5	5.9	6.8
Group II: normal lactate						
Control	Mean	50	75	128	73	97
	±SE	2.3	4.5	4.9	2.0	4.1
Pacing	Mean		131	131	86	103
	±SE		4.1	5.0	2.1	2.7
Hand grip	Mean		91	177	99	131
	±SE		4.8	9.6	4.5	5.9
Pacing plus	Mean		131	160	102	127
hand grip	±SE		5.0	10.1	3.8	6.8

studies with hand grip: Group I—Abnormal lactate (nine patients): Group II—
METABOLISM DURING ISOMETRIC HAND GRIP TEST, British Heart

TTI (mmHg sec/ min)	Triple product HRxSPx ET	LVET (msec)	Myocardial arteriovenous O_2 diff. (vol. %)	Myocardial O_2 extraction ratio (%)
2591	3206	320	12.82	65
134	183	7	0.36	2.74
3165	4019	220	13.11	66
191	189	9	0.49	2.29
3779	4484	300	13.89	69
172	211	9	0.44	1.47
4299	5347	240	13.9	68
269	361	8	0.87	3.04
2393	2894	300	11.76	64
147	198	5	0.44	1.51
3303	3861	240	11.31	60
241	193	2	0.47	2.05
3807	4662	290	12.36	65
246	338	5	0.53	1.56
4146	4962	240	12.04	65
230	322	8	0.58	2.31

there is often an increase in left ventricular end-diastolic pressure; while the left ventricular end-diastolic volume diminished, end-systolic volume increased and hence ejection fraction diminished.

Contraindications to isometric hand grip[6]: Although the isometric hand grip test is easily done at the bedside and in the cardiac catheterization laboratory, there are several contraindications to this test: 1) acute or recent myocardial infarction; 2) severe arterial hypertension; 3) symptomatic patients with cerebral vascular accident; 4) cerebral vascular malfunction; 5) serious cardiac arrhythmias; and 6) in the elderly (especially moderate or severe degree of hand grip).

References

1. Krayenbuehl, H. P., Rutishauser, W., Schoenbeck, M. and Amende, I. Evaluation of left ventricular function from isovolumic pressure measurements during isometric exercise. Am. J. Cardiol. 29:323, 1972.
2. Donald, K. W., Lind, A. R., McNicol, G. W., Humphreys, P. W., Taylor, S. H., Staunton, H. P. Cardiovascular responses to sustained (static) contractions. Circ. Res. (Suppl. I) 20:1–15, 1967.
3. Helfant, R. H., De Villa, M. A. and Meister, S. G. Effect of sustained isometric hand grip exercise on left ventricular performance. Circulation 44:982, 1971.
4. Koviwitz, C., Parmley, W. W., Donoso, R., Marcus, H., Ganz, W., and Swan, H. J. C. Effects of isometric exercise on cardiac performance—The grip test. Circulation 44:994, 1971.

5. Nakhjavan, F. K., Natarajan, G., Smith, A. M., Dratch, M. and Goldberg, H. Myocardial lactate metabolism during isometric hand grip test. Comparison with pacing tachycardia. Br. Heart J. 37:79, 1975.
6. Nutter, D. O., Schland, R. C. and Hurst, J. W. Isometric exercise and the cardiovascular system. Modern Concepts Cardiovasc. Dis. 41:11, 1972.
7. Lindquist, V. A. Y., Spangler, R. D., Blount, S. G., Jr. A comparison between the effects of dynamic and isometric exercise as evaluated by the systolic time intervals in normal man. Am. Heart J. 85:227, 1973.
8. Krayenbuehl, H. P., Schoenbeck, M., Rutishauser, W. and Wirz, P. Abnormal segmental contraction velocity in coronary artery disease produced by isometric exercise and atrial pacing. Am. J. Cardiol. 35:785, 1975.
9. Flessas, A. P., Connelly, G. P., Handa, S., Tilney, C. R., Kloster, C. K., Rimmer, R. H., Jr., Keefe, J. F., Klein, M. D. and Ryan, T. J. Effects of isometric exercise on the end-diastolic pressure, volumes and function of the left ventricle in man. Circulation 35:839, 1976.

3

Pacing Tachycardia as a
Stress Test

Pacing tachycardia, usually by right atrial pacing (RAP), is a commonly used stress test in most cardiac catheterization laboratories. Because of its safety, ease of performance and reproducibility, it has gained wide popularity, especially in patients with coronary artery disease. The physiological effects of pacing are thoroughly investigated and its value as a diagnostic test is well established.

Hemodynamic effects of pacing tachycardia: Increasing the heart rate by right atrial pacing over a wide range (80–120 beats/min) does not cause any significant change in cardiac output.[1] Indeed stroke volume diminishes as expected. However, when the heart rate is increased further (approximately 150 beats/min) a small reduction in cardiac output may occur. Studies by Sonnenblick et al.[2] have shown that the force of contraction does not change significantly with pacing tachycardia although the velocity of contraction increases. Hence the Bowditch effect is different in humans as compared to other species.

Although atrial contribution to cardiac output in normal hearts is only moderately significant and is on the order of 26 per cent,[3] it may be of particular importance in patients with poorly contracting myocardium or in patients with a low compliant ventricle such as in aortic stenosis. Figure III-1 demonstrates the effect of atrial contribution to cardiac output as reflected in the systemic arterial pressure in a patient with heart block and a ventricular demand pacemaker. A significant reduction in systemic arterial pressure secondary to a diminution in stroke volume occurs when the atrial contraction does not have an optimal relation to the ventricular contraction.

Technique of right atrial pacing: Generally, right atrial pacing as a stress test is performed as part of the cardiac catheterization procedure. If a venous catheter is already in position (usually in the coronary sinus for myocardial metabolic studies or in the pulmonary artery), a small No. 4F or 5F electrode catheter may be used through the same vein, or a separate vein may be used. The tip of the catheter is positioned in the right atrium where stable pacing can be achieved. Some investigators use a Goodale type bipolar electrode catheter* for coronary sinus catheterization and pacing by the same catheter. The intensity of the stimulus is gradually increased until the atrium is responsive to each stimulus. It should be mentioned that a strong stimulus current in the lateral atrial wall may stimulate the phrenic nerve and cause contractions of the diaphragm. Generally the pacing rate is increased by increments of 10 beats every 2–5 minutes until a rate of 150/min or more is reached, or the patient experiences angina, or Wenckebach atrioventricular block occurs. Because of the latter, ventricular pacing may have to be performed instead of atrial pacing. Pacing protocol may be varied according to the clinical situation and the information sought. In addition to the electrocardiogram, we generally monitor aortic or brachial arterial pressures during pacing. We have not had any complications in over several hundred pacing studies except for a few episodes of transient atrial fibrillation. If two

---

* Gorlin electrode catheter, U.S.C.I. Co.

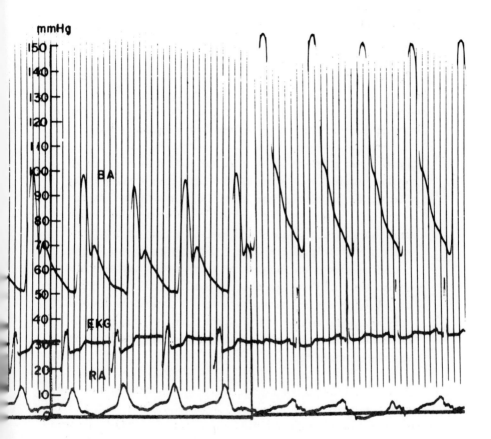

Fig. III-1. The effect of atrial contribution to cardiac output as reflected in the brachial arterial pressure in a patient with ventricular demand pacemaker. During paced beats, when the atrial contraction occurs at the time when mitral and tricuspid valves are closed, brachial arterial pressure is markedly diminished. Note the "Cannon" waves in right atrial pressure tracing.

catheters are used in the same vein and the procedure has been of long duration, the catheters should be removed simultaneously after completion of the studies since blood clots may be formed between the two catheters.

Pacing in heart disease: There are generally three types of heart disease in which atrial pacing is particularly useful: 1) coronary artery disease; 2) valvular heart disease; 3) conduction abnormalities (which will be discussed in a separate chapter).

1) Coronary artery disease: Atrial pacing has been particularly useful in the study of patients with coronary artery disease. By increasing the heart rate, myocardial oxygen demand is increased (as estimated by an increase in tension time index which is calculated as the product of heart rate × mean systolic pressure). Since the only major variable in pacing studies is an increase in heart rate, a reproducible angina threshold[4] is often obtained which is especially useful in the follow-up hemodynamic study of patients with coronary artery disease, to determine the effects of various medications or postoperatively for evaluation of the results of revascularization surgery.

As was mentioned previously, pacing tachycardia causes a reduction in stroke volume which results in a diminution in left ventricular end-diastolic volume and pressure (LVEDP) according to the Frank-Starling mechanism. However, in patients with coronary artery disease, LVEDP may increase, which is an abnormal finding. The elevation of LVEDP during pacing may be due to changes in compliance or secondary to "contracture" of the ischemic part of the myocardium[5] or to an impairment of ventricular relaxation.[6] It should be mentioned that accurate measurement of LVEDP with the usual fluid-filled catheter-manometer systems during rapid heart rates may be difficult, and catheter tipped micromanometers are superior in this regard.

Also, prolongation of PR interval during pacing by itself may influence LVEDP as compared to the control LVEDP during the patient's spontaneous heart rate.

Post-pacing studies: When atrial pacing is suddenly interrupted, the post-pacing changes in LVEDP yield useful information. The first post-pacing beat, the maximal post-pacing beat, or an average of several post-pacing beats may be used. In our study of 34 patients (17 patients with coronary artery disease and 17 control patients with normal coronary arteriogram), the maximal post-pacing LVEDP was found to be more useful than the first post-pacing, or the average of 20 post-pacing beats, in distinguishing patients with coronary artery disease from the control group. The post-pacing changes in LVEDP are most likely due to alterations in myocardial compliance. Figure III-2 shows the post-pacing LVEDP in a patient with coronary artery disease. In 17 patients with coronary artery disease, mean maximal post-pacing LVEDP was 23.30 mmHg ± 2.15 SEM as compared to 13.12 mmHg ± 0.93 SEM in the control group (P < 0.01) (Fig. III-3). In none of the patients in the control group was the maximal post-pacing LVEDP higher than 20 mmHg. The increase in post-pacing LVEDP was 10.6 mmHg ± 1.4 SEM in patients with two vessel disease, and 13.8 mmHg ± 2.3 SEM in patients with three vessel disease.

Ventricular function curves during pacing: By relating left ventricular end-diastolic pressure to left ventricular stroke work (LVSW) during pacing, "pacing ventricular function curves" are obtained which have been useful in differentiating patients with normal from abnormal myocardial function.[7,8] Figure III-4 shows schematically the pacing left ventricular function curves in patients with normal vs. abnormal myocardial function. In patients with normal myocardial function, LVSW increases, while LVEDP decreases. In patients with abnormal myocardial function, LVSW changes slightly, while there is a significant increase

50

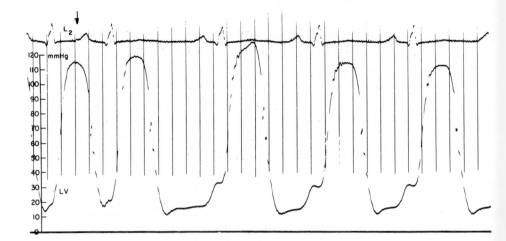

Fig. III-2. Post-pacing left ventricular pressure in a patient with coronary artery disease. Right atrial pacing was abruptly discontinued at arrow. Note the marked increase in LVEDP in post-pacing period.

in LVEDP. In addition, as is shown by Linhart,[9] in patients with coronary artery disease, pacing ventricular function curves are abnormal in 90 per cent of the patients during angina and in 60 per cent in the absence of angina. Also, abnormalities of myocardial contraction may appear or become aggravated during pacing-induced myocardial ischemia as shown by left ventriculograms obtained during pacing.[10]

Angina and myocardial metabolic changes during pacing: Pacing tachycardia is a reliable stress test for inducing angina and electrocardiographic changes in patients with coronary artery disease. As was mentioned previously, angina is usually repro-

Fig. III-3. Left ventricular end-
diastolic pressure before and after pacing tachycardia in a group of patients
with coronary artery disease and in a
control group. Note the significant difference in LVEDP between the two
groups, especially in the post-pacing
period.

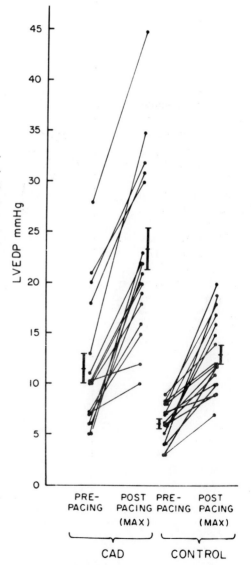

Fig. III-4. Schematic representation of left ventricular function curve during pacing by relating LVEDP to LVSW. The patients with normal myocardium have an increase in LVSW with a decrease in LVEDP. In contrast, an abnormal myocardial response is represented by a large increase in LVEDP and a small change in LVSW.

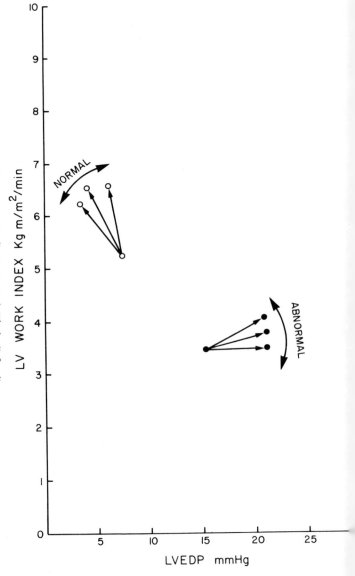

ducible at the same pacing rate and usually disappears shortly after interruption, of pacing. Pacing studies are therefore extremely useful in various investigations.

Abnormalities of myocardial metabolism evidenced by lactate production or less than 10 per cent extraction are often shown in patients with coronary artery disease in whom angina is produced by pacing tachycardia. These abnormalities are more often seen in patients with three vessel disease, since the area of ischemia is more diffuse and thus well represented by coronary sinus sampling. In patients with the syndrome of "angina and normal coronary arteriograms," myocardial lactate abnormalities are present in approximately 30 to 40 per cent of patients. In addition, myocardial lactate abnormalities are present in 30 per cent of patients with prolapsing mitral leaflet syndrome who also often have chest pain with normal coronary arteriograms.[11,12]

2) Pacing tachycardia in valvular heart disease: The most common use of pacing tachycardia in valvular heart disease is in the study of mitral stenosis. Because of an increase in the resistance to flow at the stenosed mitral valve, the duration of diastole is of particular importance in maintaining the flow. When diastole is shortened during tachycardia, left atrial pressure must rise to maintain the flow across the mitral valve. In our studies on the effects of tachycardia, catecholamine stimulation and exercise in mitral stenosis, tachycardia caused an increase in mitral valve gradient and left atrial pressure with no significant change in cardiac output and a reduction in diastolic filling period[13] (Fig. III-5). The hemodynamic effects of tachycardia in aortic regurgitation are demonstrated by Judge et al.[14] (Fig. III-6). They have shown that tachycardia causes a significant reduction in the left ventricular end-diastolic pressure, left ventricular end-diastolic volume and total stroke volume. Forward car-

Fig. III-5. Pacing tachycardia in patients with mitral stenosis (compared with exercise and isoproterenol). During pacing, there is a shortening of diastolic filling period (A) while mitral valve gradient increases with no significant change in cardiac output (B). (From Nakhjavan et al. Hemodynamic effects of exercise, catecholamine stimulation and tachycardia in mitral stenosis and sinus rhythm at comparable heart rates. Am. J. Cardiol. 23:659, 1969.)

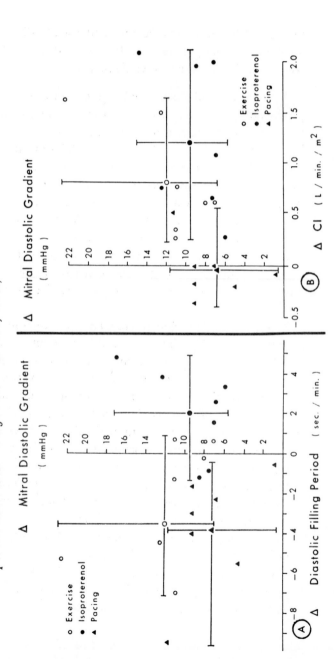

Fig. III-6. The effect of tachycardia by right atrial pacing in patients with aortic regurgitation. The open bar in the center represents the normal range for LVEDP. (From Judge et al. Circulation 44: 55, 1971.)

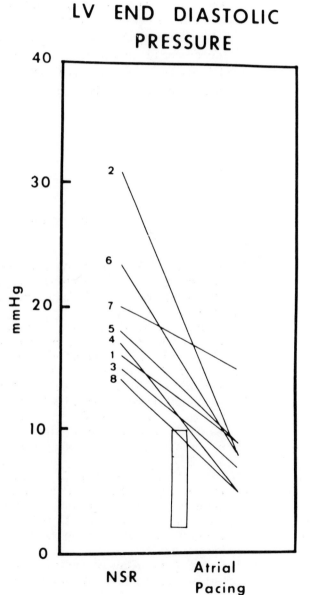

LV END DIASTOLIC PRESSURE

diac output increased with pacing but the regurgitant flow per minute is not changed significantly.

Atrial pacing in valvular aortic stenosis causes a small reduction or no change in the transvalvular aortic gradient, while stroke volume and LVEDP diminish with no significant change in cardiac output.[15]

References

1. Ross, J., Jr., Linhart, J. W. and Braunwald, E. Effects of changing heart rate in man by electrical stimulation of the right atrium. Studies at rest, during exercise, and with isoproterenol. Circulation 32:549, 1965.
2. Sonnenblick, E. H., Morrow, A. G. and Williams, J. F., Jr. Effects of heart rate on the dynamics of force development in the intact human ventricle. Circulation 33:945, 1966.
3. Stott, D. K., Marpole, D. G. F., Bristow, J. D., Kloster, F. E. and Griswold, H. E. The role of left atrial transport in aortic and mitral stenosis. Circulation 41:1031, 1970.
4. Sowton, G. E., Cross, B. D., Frick, M. H. and Balcon, R. Measurement of the angina threshold using atrial pacing. A new technic for the study of angina pectoris. Cardiovasc. Res. 301, 1967.
5. Barry, W. H., Brooker, J. Z., Alderman, E. L. and Harrison, D. C. Changes in diastolic stiffness and tone of the left ventricle during angina pectoris. Circulation 51:49, 1974.
6. McLaurin, L. P., Rolett, E. L. and Grossman, W. Impaired left ventricular relaxation during pacing-induced ischemia. Am. J. Cardiol. 32:751, 1973.
7. Parker, J. O., Khya, F. and Case, R. B. Analysis of left ventricular function by atrial pacing. Circulation 43:241, 1971.

8. Linhart, J. W. Pacing-induced changes in stroke volume in the evaluation of myocardial function. Circulation 43:253, 1971.
9. Linhart, J. W. Atrial pacing in coronary artery disease, including preinfarction angina and postoperative studies. Am. J. Cardiol. 30:603, 1972.
10. Dwyer, E. M., Jr. Left ventricular pressure-volume alterations and regional disorders of contraction during myocardial ischemia induced by atrial pacing. Circulation 42:1111, 1970.
11. Natarajan, G., Nakhjavan, F. K., Kahn, D., Yazdanfar, S., Sahibzada, W., Khawaja, F. and Goldberg, H. Myocardial metabolic studies in prolapsing mitral leaflet syndrome. Circulation 52:1105, 1975.
12. Nakhjavan, F. K., Natarajan, G., Seshachary, P. and Goldberg, H. The relationship between prolapsing mitral leaflet syndrome and angina and normal coronary arteriograms. Chest 70:706, 1976.
13. Nakhjavan, F., Katz, M., Shedrovilsky, H., Maranhao, V. and Goldberg, H. Hemodynamic effects of exercise, catecholamine stimulation and tachycardia in mitral stenosis and sinus rhythm at comparable heart rates. Am. J. Cardiol. 23:659, 1969.
14. Judge, T. P., Kennedy, J. W., Bennett, L. J., Wills, R. E., Murray, J. A., Blackmon, J. R. Quantitative hemodynamic effects of heart rate in aortic regurgitation. Circulation 44:355, 1971.
15. Linhart, J. W. Hemodynamic consequences of pacing-induced changes in heart rate in valvular aortic stenosis. Circulation 45:300, 1972.

4

Pacing Tachycardia for Detection of Conduction System Abnormalities

A variety of pacing techniques have been used in the study of the cardiac conduction system. Two of the most widely applied of these consist of constant pacing at rates in excess of the prevailing sinus rate (over-drive), and the application of precisely timed extrastimuli (extrastimulus technique). Using these two techniques, considerable experience has been gathered in recent years in the evaluation of sinus node function, A-V conduction, and in the determination of cardiac refractory periods.

I. Detection of Abnormalities of the Sinus Node Function:

Sinus recovery time[1-3]: Since at present it is not possible to record the sinus node potentials directly by intra-cardiac electrocardiography, sinus node malfunction may be assessed by information obtained from pacing tachycardia. The right atrium is paced at rates of 60–150/min for periods of one to two minutes, and the pacing is then suddenly discontinued. It is important to record the right atrial potentials by an electrode catheter in addition to the surface electrocardiograms. In practice, pacing is performed at different rates—starting above the patient's control

59

heart rate. It should be kept in mind that at faster heart rates the sinus node may not be penetrated by 1:1 conduction because of possible sino-atrial block; hence it is of particular importance to perform the test at slower paced rates. Sinus recovery time (SRT) is determined by measuring the interval between the last atrial paced beat and the first sinus beat or ectopic beat. The latter measurement does not represent the true SRT. Since SRT varies with the control sinus rate, the corrected SRT is often used: corrected SRT (SRT$_c$) = SRT − control P − P interval. Figure IV-1 shows a patient with sick sinus syndrome (see legend). In Narula's laboratory, SRT$_c$ ranged from 100–525 msec (mean 260 ± 95 msec).[3] In the study reported by Gupta et al.,[4] the SRT$_c$ in control subjects ranged from 0 to 375 msec (mean 210 ± 131). In 17 patients with sick sinus syndrome, SRT$_c$ was prolonged (480 to 5,690 msec) in 6 patients, and normal in 11. Hence a normal SRT does not rule out sick sinus syndrome. When pacing studies for SRT measurement are repeated after intravenous administration of 0.6 to 2 mg atropine, abnormal response may be detected in some patients who had normal SRT during the control state before the administration of atropine.[4]

Premature atrial stimulation for detection of sinus node malfunction: Premature atrial stimulation is another method used for evaluation of sinus node function.[5,6] In this technique, a premature atrial stimulus is delivered during atrial diastole. Late in atrial diastole, the premature atrial depolarization is followed by a full compensatory pause which indicates that the sinus pacemaker was not discharged (non-reset). Early in atrial diastole, the premature atrial stimulus is followed by a less than compensatory pause (reset). Thus, two zones are identified, i.e., non-reset and reset zones (Figs. IV-2 and 3). Sino-atrial conduction time is calculated as one-half the difference between A$_2$ − A$_3$ and A$_1$ − A$_1$ intervals during the zone of reset, where A$_2$ is the extra stimulus, A$_3$ is the first spontaneous sinus beat following A$_2$,

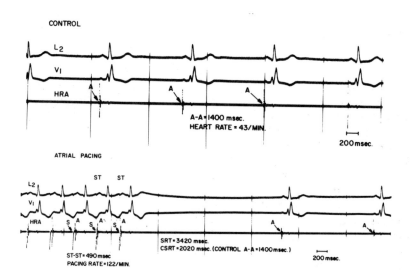

Fig. IV-1. Sick sinus syndrome. Lead II, V_1 and high right atrial electrogram are simultaneously recorded. A) Control tracing. B) After sudden cessation of pacing, there is a long pause. Corrected sinus recovery time is markedly prolonged (2020 msec).

and $A_1 - A_1$ is the spontaneous sinus cycle. Points falling in the last third of zone II (adjacent to zone I) are used to measure $A_2A_3 - A_1A_1$. There are several assumptions in the above mentioned calculations:

1. The sinus automaticity does not change and there is no shift in the sinus pacemaker
2. The extra stimulus is penetrating the sinus node and resetting it
3. The antegrade and retrograde conduction times are equal.

Sino-atrial conduction time is measured as the average of several points in the reset zone closest to the non-reset zone. In some patients, reset may never be seen due to marked prolongation of the sino-atrial conduction, and therefore the sinus impulse in its

62

Fig. IV-2. Schematic representation of sinus nodal response and the two zones. A_1A_3 interval is plotted against A_1A_2 interval. A_1A_3 is the interval between the last spontaneous sinus beat and the first spontaneous sinus beat following extra-stimulus (A_2). A_1A_2 is the interval between the last spontaneous sinus beat and the extra-stimulus. Sino-atrial conduction time is measured from the mean of several points in zone II, adjacent to zone I.

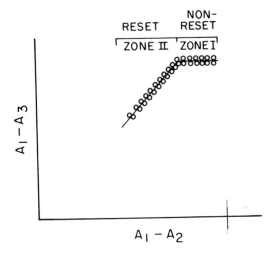

passage to the atrium collides with the extra stimulus. Thus SACT cannot always be determined by this technique. The reported normal range for sino-atrial conduction time varies according to different investigators: 40–70 msec,[7] 39.5 − 97.5 msec,[8] 28.5–115.5 msec,[9] and 40–153 msec.[10]

It should be mentioned that measurement of sinus recovery time by rapid atrial pacing and sino-atrial conduction time by premature atrial stimulation identify two different mechanisms. Sinus recovery time is a measure of automaticity of the sinus node, while sino-atrial conduction time is a measure of perinodal conduction. This is probably why the correlation between sinus recovery time and sino-atrial conduction time is not good.

Atrial pacing for measurement of sino-atrial conduction time: Recently Narula and colleagues[11] have used a new and simple technique for measurement of SACT. In this technique, high right atrial pacing is performed as a train of eight beats at rates which are slightly faster than the sinus rate ($\leqslant$10 beats/min).

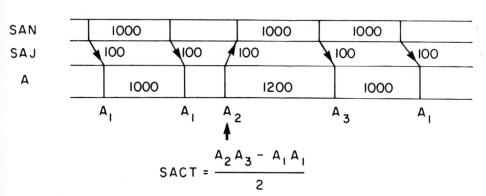

Fig. IV-3. Schematic demonstration of premature atrial stimulation for assessment of sino-atrial conduction time. A_1A_1 is the spontaneous sinus cycle. A_2 is the premature extra stimulus. A_3 is the first sinus beat following A_2. SAN: Sino-atrial node; SAJ: Sino-atrial junction; A: Atrium; SACT: Sino-atrial conduction time.

The interval between the last paced atrial electrogram and the first escape atrial electrogram of sinus origin is measured (AP − A). SACT by this technique is measured as the difference between AP–A minus A_1A_1 (mean sinus cycle length). Since this interval represents the conduction into and out of the sinus node, it should be divided by two. The pacing rate should be only slightly faster than the sinus rate, as mentioned above, otherwise the automaticity of the sinus node will be suppressed and SACT cannot be measured. This new technique is much simpler to apply than the extra stimulus method and also requires less time.

II. Detection of Conduction Abnormalities of the Atrio-Ventricular-His-Purkinje System: Because of decremental conduction in atrio-ventricular node, Wenckebach type I block is frequently seen in pacing rates above 130/min. However, the occurrence of Wenckebach type A-V block below 130/min is probably abnormal. His bundle electrograms reveal that progressive increase in conduction delay is localized in A-V node as manifested by prolongation of the A-H interval (Fig. IV-4). The occurrence of Wenckebach type block in His-Purkinje system as manifested by prolongation of H-V interval in His bundle electrograms is rare even in patients with diseased His-Purkinje system. Figure IV-5 shows a patient with left axis deviation and right bundle branch block in whom pacing tachycardia caused Wenckebach of the remaining fascicle (posterior fascicle of the left bundle—see legend).

III. Pacing for Measurement of Refractory Periods of Conduction Tissues: The phenomenon of refractoriness is common to all excitable tissues and is an important determinant of im-

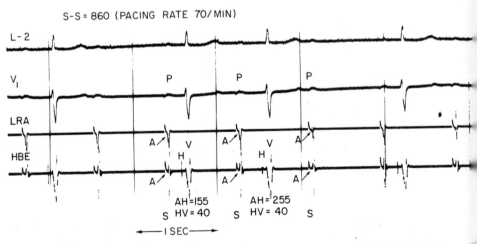

Fig. IV-4. Wenckebach type block during pacing at the rate of 70/min. There is progressive increase in A-H intervals with subsequent block above the His bundle. LRA: Low right atrial electrogram; HBE: His bundle electrogram; S: Stimulus artefact.

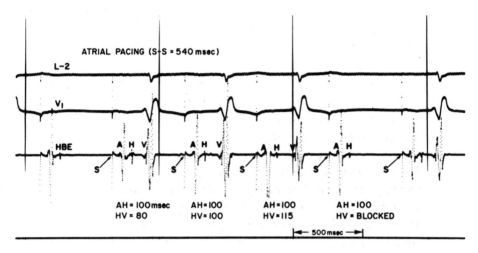

Fig. IV-5. Wenckebach type block in the posterior fascicle of the left bundle. The patient has left axis deviation and right bundle branch block (bi-fascicular block). With atrial pacing at the rate of 110/min, there is progressive increase in HV interval with subsequent block (4:3 Wenckebach block) while A-H interval remains constant (120 msec).

pulse propagation. Since the atrio-ventricular conduction system of the heart is composed of various elements (the atria, the AV node, the His-Purkinje system, and the ventricular muscle) with different electrical properties, conduction of the sinus impulse to the ventricles is influenced by the refractoriness or the responsiveness of each of these various elements. The known differences in the refractory periods of these components of the conduction system have been used to explain the occurrence of arrhythmias such as AV block, various types of bundle branch block and aberrant conduction. Until recently, our understanding of the cardiac refractory periods had been based on data derived from experimental animals and isolated tissues. However, with the advent of His bundle electrocardiography, it has become possible to study cardiac refractory periods in the human heart under a variety of conditions.[12]

Technique:

In the most widely used technique for the determination of cardiac refractory periods, the atria are paced at a rate just above the spontaneous sinus rate (in order to eliminate the influence of sinus arrhythmia, premature beats, and escape beats on the refractory periods), and single premature atrial stimuli (test stimuli) are applied at various points in the cardiac cycle. Since the test stimulus may alter the refractory period in several subsequent cycles,[13] the stimulator is programmed to deliver the test stimulus after every 8th or 10th beat of the basic rhythm. The use of a programmable stimulator facilitates rapid and accurate adjustment of the timing of the test stimulus so that the entire diastolic cycle can be scanned with relative ease. In the typical study, the test stimulus (A2) is initially applied late in diastole and then at decreasing coupling intervals relative to the preceding basic drive stimulus (A1) until the atrium or the AV node becomes refractory. One or more surface electrocardiographic leads, intra atrial, and a His bundle electrocardiogram are simultaneously recorded to enable the detection and localization of delay or block in conduction of the test stimulus.

A variety of terms have been used to describe cardiac refractory periods determined in this manner. Two of the most commonly used expressions of refractory periods are: *the effective refractory period* and *the functional refractory period*. The effective refractory period begins when a propagated response can no longer be evoked at a site distal to the tissue being studied. The functional refractory period refers to the minimum interval between successive responses propagated through the tissue being studied. These definitions of the effective and functional refractory periods may be illustrated by examining the sequence of events during the application of test stimuli as described above (Fig. IV-6). As the interval between the basic drive stimulus (A_1) and the test stimulus (A_2) is decreased, the interval between the corresponding His bundle responses (H_1 and H_2) initially decreases in proportion to the decrease in the A_1A_2 interval. Because of increasing delay in the AV nodal propagation of the test stimulus, a point is reached where the H_1H_2 interval begins to exceed the A_1A_2 interval. With further decreases in the A_1A_2 interval, the H_1H_2 interval continues to decrease until a certain point in diastole when the H_1H_2 interval begins to increase. The A_1A_2 interval at which the shortest H_1H_2 interval occurs defines the functional refractory period of the AV node. If the A_1A_2 interval is further decreased, A_2 eventually fails to be conducted to the His bundle. The longest A_1A_2 interval at which A_2 is not conducted (propagated) to the His bundle defines the effective refractory period of the AV node.

The following is a list of definitions of refractory periods commonly used in electrophysiology literature:

a. Effective refractory periods (ERP)

The AV node: The ERP of the AV node is the longest coupling interval (A_1A_2) at which the test stimulus (A_2) fails to conduct to the His bundle.

The His-Purkinje system: The ERP of the His-Purkinje system is the longest H_1H_2 interval at which H_2 is not conducted to the ventricles.

The bundle branches: The longest H_1H_2 interval at which H_2 gives rise to the appropriate bundle branch block configuration.

b. Functional refractory periods (FRP)

The AV node: The FRP of the AV node is the shortest H_1H_2 interval achieved during the application of progressively earlier test stimuli to the atrium.

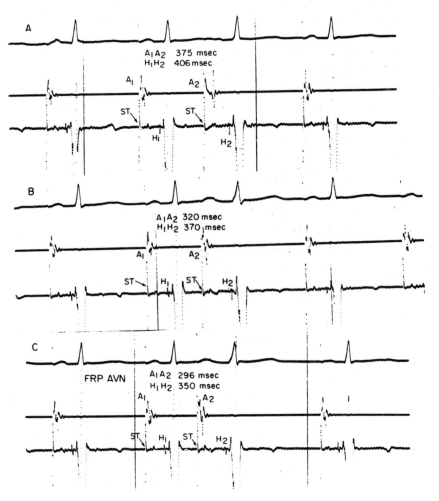

Fig. IV-6. The extra-stimulus study for measurement of refractory periods. A_1A
is the coupling interval of the extra-stimulus. Stimulus artefact is indicated by a
rows. When A_1A_2 is shortened to 296 msec (Panel C) the functional refractor
period (FRP) of the atrioventricular node (AVN) is reached (where $H_1H_2 = 3$
msec is the shortest interval). By shortening the A_1A_2 interval (panel D, A_1A_2

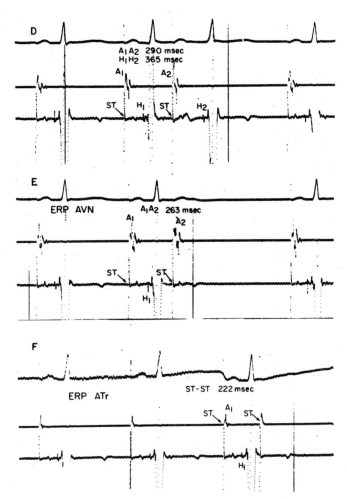

90 msec), H_1H_2 becomes longer (365 msec). By shortening the coupling interval further, effective refractory period (ERP) of the atrioventricular node is reached (panel E, $A_1A_2 = 263$ msec) where A_2 is not conducted to His bundle. By shortening the coupling interval further, ERP of the atrium is reached (panel F, ST–ST = 222 msec) where the extra-stimulus does not stimulate the atrium.

The His-Purkinje system: The FRP of the His-Purkinje system is the shortest interval between successive ventricular responses (V_1V_2) propagated from the His bundle.

The foregoing technique has been widely applied to determine the refractory periods of the atrium, AV node, and the His-Purkinje system in the human heart. It has been shown that the responses of the human heart to changes in cycle length are generally similar to those described in experimental animals.[14] The changes in the refractory period induced by changes in the cycle length are most marked in the His-Purkinje system and least prominent in the AV node. At heart rates between 70 and 100/min the AV nodal refractory period ranges between 250 and 365 msec.

An important application of this technique to determine refractory periods has been in the study of patients with pre-excitation. Since the initiation and the perpetuation of tachycardias in pre-excitation depends on the disparity between the refractory periods of the AV nodal and the accessory pathways, it would appear that patients prone to develop tachycardias could be identified. Further, it might be possible to minimize the disparity between the refractory periods of the AV nodal and accessory pathways by the administration of certain drugs that selectively influence the refractory period of the AV nodal or the accessory pathway, thereby preventing the occurrence of tachycardias. At present, these expectations have not been fulfilled, and more work needs to be done in this area.

References

1. Narula, S., Samet, P. and Javier, R. P. Significance of the sinus-node recovery time. Circulation 45:140, 1972.
2. Mandel, W. J., Hayakawa, H., Allen, H. N., Danzig, R. and Kermaier, A. I. Assessment of sinus node function in patients with the sick sinus syndrome. Circulation 46:761, 1972.

3. Narula, O. S. Disorders of sinus node function: Electrophysiologic evaluation. *In* His Bundle Electrocardiography and Clinical Electrophysiology (Narula, O. S.) F. A. Davis Co., 1975, p. 275.
4. Gupta, P. K., Lichstein, E., Chadda, K. D. and Badui, E. Appraisal of sinus nodal recovery time in patients with sick sinus syndrome. Am. J. Cardiol. 34:254, 1974.
5. Strauss, H. C., Saroff, A. L., Bigger, J. W., Jr. and Giardina, E. G. V. Premature atrial stimulation as a key to the understanding of sinoatrial conduction in man. Circulation 47:86, 1973.
6. Dhingra, R. C., Amat-Y-Leon, F., Wyndham, C., Deedwania, P. C., Wu, D., Denes, P. and Rosen, K. M. Clinical significance of prolonged sinoatrial conduction time. Circulation 55:8, 1977.
7. Steinbeck, G. and Luderitz, B. Comparative study of sinoatrial conduction time and sinus node recovery time. Br. Heart J. 37:956, 1975.
8. Masini, G., Dianda, R. and Graziina, A. Analysis of sinoatrial conduction in man using premature atrial stimulation. Cardiovasc. Res. 9:498, 1975.
9. Engle, T. R., Bond, R. C. and Schaal, S. F. First degree sinoatrial heart block: Sinoatrial block in the sick-sinus syndrome. Am. Heart J. 91:303, 1976.
10. Dhingra, R. C., Wyndham, C., Amat-Y-Leon, F., Denes, P., Wu, D. and Rosen, K. M. Sinus nodal responses to atrial extrastimuli in patients without apparent sinus node disease. Am. J. Cardiol. 36:445, 1975.
11. Narula, O. S., Shantha, N., Vasquez, M., Towne, W. D. and Linhart, J. W. A new method for measurement of sinoatrial conduction time. Circulation 58:706, 1978.
12. Damato, A. N., Caracta, A. R., Akhtar, M. and Lau, S. H. The effects of commonly used cardiovascular drugs on AV conduction and refractoriness. *In* His Bundle Electrocardiography and Clinical Electrophysiology (Narula, O. S.) F. A. Davis Co., 1975, p. 105.
13. Denes, P., Wu, D., Dhingra, R., Pietras, R. J. and Rosen, K. M. The effects of cycle length on cardiac refractory periods in man. Circulation 49:32, 1976.
14. Mendez, C., Gruhzit, C. C. and Moe, G. K. Influence of cycle length upon refractory period of auricles, ventricles and A-V node in the dog. Am. J. Physiol. 184:287, 1956.

5

Angiographic Studies as a Stress Test

Angiographic studies, particularly left ventriculography (LVG), have been used to assess the left ventricular function. Since rapid infusion of contrast material into the systemic circulation acts as a volume load on the heart, ventricular function may be estimated by comparing the post-left ventriculographic data with the control state.

Hemodynamic effects of left ventriculography: Left ventriculography is usually performed by rapid injection of a large volume (40–60 ml) of contrast material into the cavity of the left ventricle. The hemodynamic effects of left ventriculography are described by several investigators.[1-11] After left ventriculography, cardiac output, stroke volume and stroke work increase. Left ventricular end-diastolic and most often systolic pressures increase and the peripheral resistance diminishes. On the other hand, contrast material has a depressant effect on myocardial contractility. The above mentioned changes last for approximately 15–20 minutes. Except for decreased myocardial contractility, which is attributed to the high sodium content of the radiopaque material, other effects are generally due to volume loading of the circulation. Because of hyperosmolarity of the contrast material, a fluid shift from intracellular compartment to intravascular compartment occurs, with subsequent hemodilution.

Post-left ventriculographic changes in left ventricular end-diastolic pressure (LVEDP): Post-LVG-LVEDP is often used as a measure of myocardial function. The increase in LVEDP after left ventriculography is well shown in patients with a low compliant heart, such as in coronary artery disease and cardiomyopathy (Fig. V-1A and B). In our laboratory, mean and maximal LVEDP in 20 beats is measured one minute after left ventriculography. As in pacing studies, maximal LVEDP was more diagnostic than mean LVEDP (measurement of the first post-LVG-LVEDP is not practical). In our laboratory we have studied 34 patients, 17 with coronary artery disease and 17 control patients. Before left ventriculography, LVEDP in the control group was 5.82 mmHg ± 0.40 (SEM) and increased to 16.59 mmHg ± 1.10 (SEM) after left ventriculography. In the CAD group, control LVEDP was 11.80 mmHg ± 1.60 (SEM) which increased to 24.90 mmMg ± 2.43 (SEM) after left ventriculography (Fig. V-2). Although there is an overlap between the two groups, an increase in LVEDP in excess of 23 mmHg or more was usually seen in patients with CAD.

Relationship between LVEDP and stroke work after LVG:

Modified left ventricular function curves may be constructed by relating LVEDP to left ventricular stroke work index (LVSWI). Studies by Cohn et al.[9] have demonstrated that in contrast to normal patients who exhibit an ascending curve, patients with coronary artery disease have a flat or depressed curve after left ventriculography. Figure V-3 shows such a curve. Since left ventriculography is performed in almost all patients who undergo cardiac catheterization studies, it constitutes a simple and practical test for assessment of myocardial function. The increase in LVEDP after left ventriculography is most likely a combined effect of volume load and myocardial depressant effect of the contrast medium.

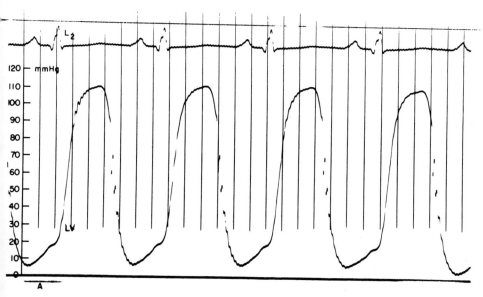

Fig. V-1. Top—Left ventricular pressure tracing during control state in a patient with coronary artery disease. Bottom—Left ventricular pressure tracing one minute after left ventriculography.

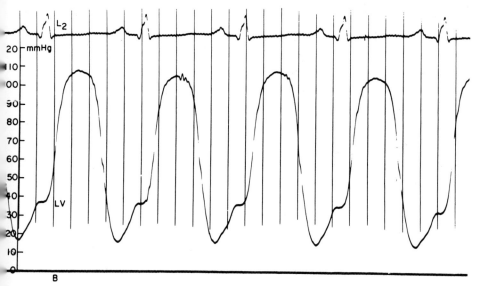

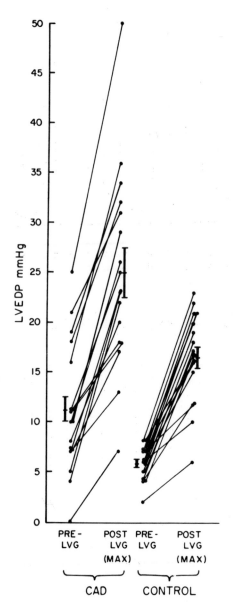

Fig. V-2. Maximal left ventricular end-diastolic pressure after left ventriculography in 17 control patients and 17 with coronary artery disease.

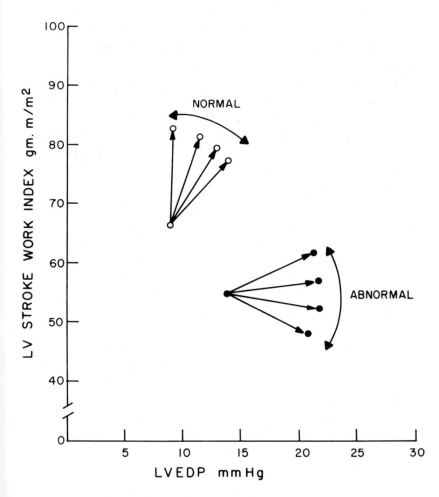

Fig. V-3. Schematic illustration of the hemodynamic effects of left ventricu-
graphy on ventricular function as represented by the relationship between left
entricular stroke work index (LVSWI) and left ventricular end-diastolic
ressure.

**Comparison of hemodynamic effects of pacing tachycardia
and left ventriculography:** Figure V-4 shows the changes in
LVEDP after pacing and left ventriculography in 34 patients
(17 with coronary artery disease and 17 control subjects) who
were studied in our laboratory. As mentioned previously, post-
pacing changes in LVEDP are generally attributed to abnormalities of myocardial function or to changes in myocardial compliance. On the other hand, left ventriculography causes significant
increases in plasma volume and depression of myocardial function, both of which affect LVEDP. Thus it appears that pacing
tachycardia has a relatively more "pure" effect on cardiovascular
function compared to left ventriculography. Pacing tachycardia
also causes angina more frequently than left ventriculography,
since the latter causes only a moderate degree of tachycardia. In
our studies, there was no relationship between the occurrence of
angina during pacing and post-pacing LVEDP. Since LVEDP
per se is not a sensitive measure of myocardial function, the
changes in LVEDP after left ventriculography or pacing tachycardia may not differentiate between the "individual" patient
with normal or abnormal myocardial function. It should be
mentioned that patients with coronary artery disease as a group
have a higher LVEDP after coronary arteriography as compared
to the control group, while there was overlap between the individual patients in the two groups. In addition, the changes in
LVEDP after left ventriculography or pacing tachycardia are not
related to ejection fraction or control resting cardiac output.

In summary, it may be stated that:

1. Pacing tachycardia and left ventriculography cause similar
directional changes in LVEDP

2. Maximal post-PT or post-LVG LVEDP is more diagnostic than mean LVEDP

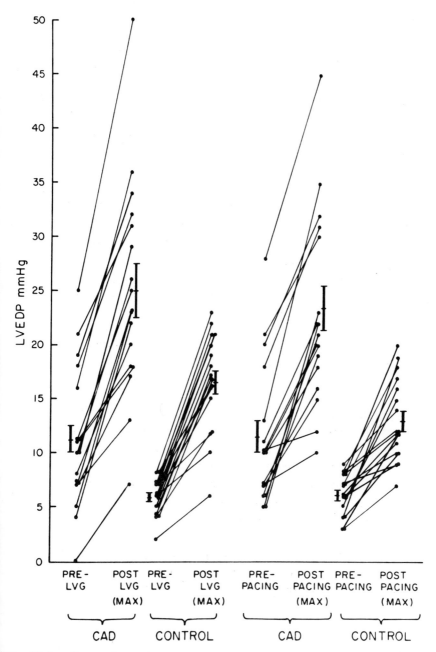

Fig. V-4. Comparison of the maximal LVEDP during the post-pacing and post-ft ventriculographic period in 17 patients with coronary artery disease and 17 ontrol patients.

3. LVEDP alone may not differentiate between individual patients in either group; however, post-LVG-LVEDP more than 23 mmHg and post-pacing-LVEDP more than 20 mmHg are usually seen in patients with coronary artery disease.

Coronary arteriography as a stress test: Some investigators have used coronary arteriography as a stress test.[12,13] In the study reported by Gensini and associates[12] and Kavanagh-Gray,[13] patients with coronary artery disease had a marked increase in LVEDP after coronary arteriography.

We have preferred left ventriculography as an angiographic stress test in our laboratory for the following reasons:

1. Control data, i.e., pressures and cardiac output, are temporally closer to angiographic data.

2. The volume of contrast material used in left ventriculography and its speed of delivery may be relatively fixed and reproducible, while in coronary cineangiography the number of injections and the amount delivered with each injection often varies from patient to patient. Hence the volume load imposed on the heart during left ventriculography is relatively uniform and the data obtained less subject to variability of the procedure.

3. During coronary arteriography, nitroglycerin or other coronary vasodilators are usually administered, and they affect the left ventricular end-diastolic pressure.

References

1. Austen, W. G., Wilcox, B. R. and Bender, H. E. Experimental studies of the cardiovascular responses secondary to the injection of angiographic agents. J. Thorac. Cardiovasc. Surg. 47:356, 1964.
2. Friesinger, G. C., Schaffer, J., Criley, J. M., Gaertner, R. A. and Ross, R. S. Hemodynamic consequences of the injection of radiopaque material. Circulation 31:730, 1965.
3. Iseri, L. T., Kaplan, M. A., Evans, M. J. and Nickel, E. D. Effect of concentrated contrast media during angiography on plasma volume and plasma osmolarity Am. Heart J. 69:154, 1965.
4. Brown, R., Rahimtoola, S. H., Davis, G. D. and Swan, H. J. C. The effect of angiocardiographic contrast medium on circulatory dynamics in man. Cardiac output during angiocardiography. Circulation 31:234, 1965.
5. Gootman, N., Rudolph, A. M. and Buckley, N. M. Effects of angiographic contrast media on cardiac function. Am. J. Cardiol. 25:59, 1970.
6. Krovetz, L. J., Simon, A. L., Levy, R. J. and Tift, W. L. Effects of angiocardiographic contrast media on left ventricular function. Bull. Johns Hopkins Med. J. 127:172, 1970.
7. Hammermeister, K. E. and Warbasse, J. R. Immediate hemodynamic effects of cardiac angiography in man. Am. J. Cardiol. 31:307, 1973.
8. Brundage, B. H. and Cheitlin, M. D. Ventricular function curves from the cardiac response to angiographic contrast: A sensitive detector of ventricular dysfunction in coronary artery disease. Am. Heart J. 88:281, 1974.
9. Cohn, P. E., Horn, H. R., Teichholz, L. E., Kreulen, T. H., Herman, M. V. and Gorlin, R. Effects of angiographic contrast medium on left ventricular function in coronary artery disease. Comparison with static and dynamic exercise. Am. J. Cardiol. 32:21, 1973.
10. Wolf, G. L., Gerlings, E. D. and Wilson, W. J. Depression of myocardial contractility induced by hypertonic coronary injections in the isolated perfused dog heart. Radiology 107:655, 1973.

11. Rahimtoola, S. H., Gau, G. T. and Raphael, M. J. Cardiac performance after diagnostic coronary arteriography. Circulation 41:537, 1970.
12. Gensini, G. G., Dubiel, J., Huntington, P. P. and Kelly, A. E. Left ventricular end-diastolic pressure before and after coronary arteriography. The value of coronary arteriography as a stress test. Am. J. Cardiol. 27:453, 1971.
13. Kavanagh-Gray, D. Left ventricular end-diastolic pressures following selective coronary arteriography. Am. Heart J. 84:629, 1972.

6

Various Maneuvers in Clinical Cardiology

Changes in posture: The changes in posture from supine to sitting or standing cause a diminution in venous return and thus cardiac output and stroke volume; and a mild degree of tachycardia.[1,2] These alterations in cardiac hemodynamics cause changes in the characteristics of heart sounds and murmurs which add important information during auscultation of the heart for differentiation of certain murmurs. For instance, the ejection systolic murmurs of aortic and pulmonic stenosis are louder in the supine position because of an increase in venous return in the flat position. On the other hand, there is no significant change in the murmur of mitral regurgitation of rheumatic origin. The late systolic murmur of prolapsing mitral leaflet becomes longer or even pansystolic in the sitting or standing position, since in this position the heart size is smaller and the mitral valve leaflet can prolapse earlier and farther into the left atrium (Fig. VI-1). In addition, the midsystolic clicks move closer to the first heart sound. Also, patients who do not have a systolic murmur in supine position may develop a murmur or click in the sitting or standing position. The murmur of idiopathic hypertrophic subaortic stenosis becomes louder in the sitting position since the degree of outflow tract obstruction becomes worse (Fig. VI-1). Because of an increase in heart volume in the supine position, the 3rd and 4th heart sounds are louder or may only be present in the supine position.

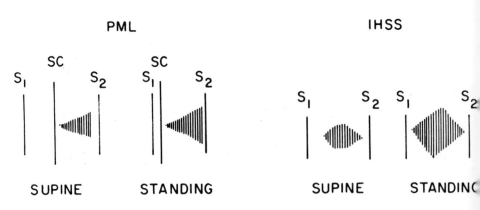

Fig. VI-1. The systolic murmur of prolapsing mitral leaflet syndrome become longer in standing position. The mid-systolic click appears earlier in systole. Th murmur of idiopathic hypertrophic subaortic stenosis (IHSS) becomes louder i standing position.

Squatting: Squatting causes an increase in venous return and cardiac output. Also, because of compression of femoral arteries, there is an increase in arterial pressure and peripheral resistance.[3] Hence the murmur of rheumatic mitral regurgitation and aortic regurgitation is increased in intensity during squatting (Fig. VI-2). Because of an increase in stroke volume, the systolic murmur of aortic and pulmonic stenosis also becomes louder. On the other hand, because of the larger ventricular volume and an increase in peripheral resistance, the murmur of idiopathic hypertrophic subaortic stenosis becomes less intense (Fig. VI-3).

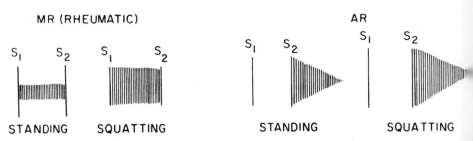

Fig. VI-2. The systolic murmur of rheumatic mitral regurgitation and the diastol murmur of aortic regurgitation become louder during squatting.

IHSS

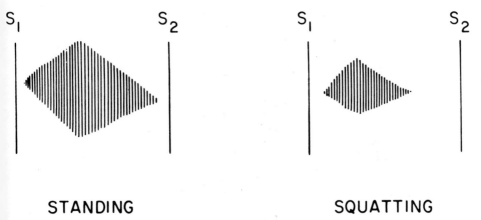

STANDING   SQUATTING

Fig. VI-3.   The systolic murmur of IHSS decreases in intensity during squatting as compared to standing.

Valsalva maneuver (Fig. VI-4): Valsalva maneuver is performed by forced expiration against a closed glottis and thus causes a significant increase in intra-thoracic pressure and therefore a diminution or interruption of venous return. It can be performed in several ways by:

1. instructing the patient to push down with the mouth closed

2. applying pressure with clenched fist on the epigastrium and instructing the patient to push against the examiner's fist with his abdomen

3. instructing the patient to blow into the tubing of a blood pressure cuff until a pressure of 40 mmHg is reached and maintained for 10 seconds. This technique of Valsalva maneuver is often used in the cardiac catheterization laboratory.

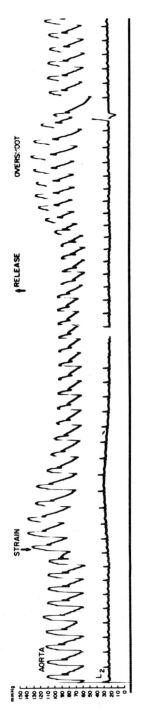

Fig. VI-4. Valsalva maneuver (see text for details).

There are four phases in the Valsalva maneuver:

Phase I: This initial phase causes a sharp rise in blood pressure which is due to a sudden increase in intra-thoracic pressure. The latter causes a diminution in venous return.

Phase II: This is the period when the intra-thoracic pressure is sustained and the venous return to the right heart is interrupted. Hence there is a progressive decrease in cardiac output, stroke volume and heart size. In idiopathic hypertrophic subaortic stenosis, because of a diminution in heart size and consequently an increase in the outflow tract obstruction, the systolic murmur becomes louder (Fig. VI-5), while the murmur of valvular aortic stenosis (Fig. VI-6), pulmonic stenosis and mitral regurgitation diminishes. The late systolic murmur of mitral valve prolapse, however, starts earlier in systole (because of a diminished heart size and early onset of prolapse and regurgitation).

Since IHSS may involve both the right and left ventricles, the right or left-sided origin of obstruction may be differentiated during phases I and II of Valsalva. The murmur of right ventricular outflow tract obstruction is increased immediately with the onset of phase I or II, since the venous return is diminished or interrupted instantly. The murmur of left ventricular outflow tract obstruction is increased after a few cardiac cycles.

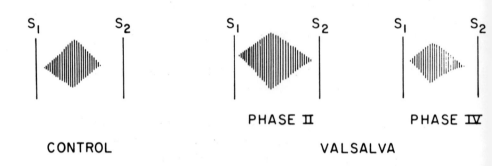

IHSS

S₁   S₂   S₁   S₂   S₁   S₂

PHASE II   PHASE IV

CONTROL   VALSALVA

Fig. VI-5. The systolic murmur of IHSS becomes louder during Phase II of Valsalva maneuver and becomes less intense during Phase IV (overshoot).

Because of a diminution in cardiac output and heart size, the third and fourth heart sounds become less intense. Since the venous return is interrupted, the ejection time of the right ventricle is shortened and thus the two components of the second heart sound become fused except in patients with atrial septal defect.

Phase III: This phase coincides with the release of straining and there is a sudden drop in the intrathoracic pressure and filling of the right ventricle. However, since the pulmonary circulation and its capacitance vessels fill up before the left ventricle, there is a further decrease in systemic pressure. Thus the murmur of right ventricular outflow tract obstruction in IHSS diminishes

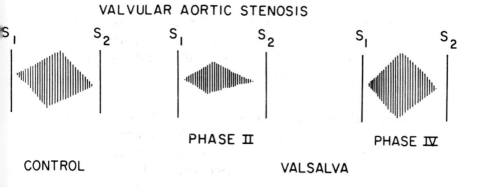

ig. VI-6. The systolic murmur of valvular aortic stenosis decreases during Phase
I of Valsalva and increases during Phase IV.

and normal splitting (which had become nar-
rowed during phase II) becomes wider except in patients with atrial septal defect.

Phase IV: During this phase, there is gradual filling of the
left ventricle and systemic pressure increases to
control and above control values (overshoot);
splitting of the second heart sound becomes
narrow, and the murmur of left ventricular
outflow obstruction of idiopathic hypertrophic
subaortic stenosis becomes less intense (Fig.
VI-5). Most of the changes in this phase are
opposite to those of phase II.

Square wave response to Valsalva maneuver: Normally during phase IV of Valsalva maneuver there is an overshoot of the
arterial pressure because of reflex vasoconstriction secondary to
diminished pulse pressure during phase III. In addition, because

of the overshoot, there is reflex bradycardia (baroreceptor stimulation). In patients with congestive heart failure and some patients with organic heart disease, the overshoot and bradycardia may not occur.[4]

Isometric hand grip (IHG): The hemodynamic effects of isometric hand grip are discussed in detail in Chapter II. Briefly, IHG causes an increase in heart rate, cardiac output and systemic arterial pressure. These hemodynamic changes cause variations in heart sounds and murmurs. Because of an increase in systemic pressure, the systolic murmur of idiopathic hypertrophic subaortic stenosis becomes less loud (Fig. VI-7), while the murmurs of mitral and aortic regurgitation increase (Fig. VI-8). Because of an increase in cardiac output and heart rate, the diastolic murmur of mitral stenosis becomes louder. In addition,

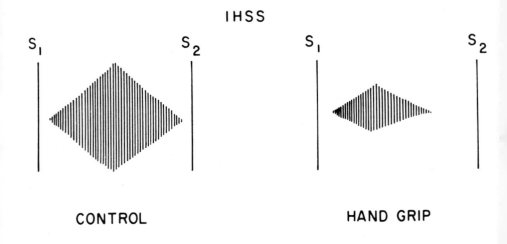

Fig. VI-7. The systolic murmur of IHSS is diminished during hand grip.

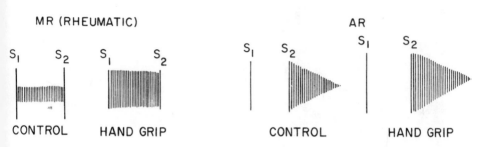

Fig. VI-8. The systolic murmur of mitral regurgitation and the diastolic murmur of aortic regurgitation increase with hand grip.

the third (S_3) and fourth (S_4) heart sounds become louder during IHG and these may be represented also on apexcardiogram or inspection of the precordium and point of maximal impulse.

References

1. McGregor, M., Adam, W. and Sekelj, P. Influence of posture on cardiac output and minute ventilation during exercise. Circ. Res. 9:1089, 1961.
2. Bevegard, S., Holmgren, A. and Jansson, B. The effect of body position on the circulation at rest and during exercise with special reference to the influence on the stroke volume. Acta Physiol. Scand. 49:279, 1960.
3. Dohan, M. C. and Criscitiello, M. Physiological and pharmacological manipulations of heart sounds and murmurs. Mod. Concepts Cardiovasc. Dis. 39:121, 1970.
4. Elisberg, E., Singian, E., Miller, G. and Katz, L. N. The effect of the Valsalva maneuver on the circulation. III. The influence of heart disease on the expected post-straining overshoot. Circulation 7:880, 1953.

7

Pharmacological Interventions

Certain pharmacological agents are often used in the cardiac catheterization laboratory for diagnostic purposes.

Nitroglycerin: In our cardiac catheterization laboratory, sublingual nitroglycerin is commonly used for diagnostic purposes.

Hemodynamic effects of nitroglycerin[1-4]: The most important action of nitroglycerin is its peripheral vasodilatation. In this regard, its action is more intense on the venous than arterial bed. Because of venous pooling, heart size, stroke volume and left ventricular end-diastolic pressure (LVEDP) diminish (Fig. VII-1). In addition, arteriolar dilatation causes a mild reduction in the arterial pressure. Because of a lower LVEDP, S_4 may disappear. Figure VII-2 shows the effect of 0.4 mg sublingual nitroglycerin on cardiac index in 45 patients (24 patients with normal heart size and 21 with enlarged hearts). In patients with normal sized heart (A) nitroglycerin caused a slight reduction in the cardiac output, while in patients with enlarged hearts (B) there was no significant change in cardiac output. Figure VII-3 shows the effect of nitroglycerin in the same group of patients on LVEDP. In patients with normal sized hearts, nitroglycerin causes a reduction in LVEDP to suboptimal filling range, while in patients with enlarged hearts who already have an elevated LVEDP, the latter is diminished towards nor-

93

94

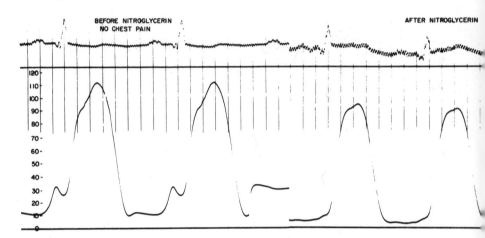

Fig. VII-1.　Effect of nitroglycerin on left ventricular end-diastolic pressure and "a" wave.

mal range. By relating LVEDP to the left ventricular stroke work, left ventricular function curve during unloading of the heart by nitroglycerin may be obtained (Fig. VII-4).

In addition, nitroglycerin can reduce the degree of mitral regurgitation. This is shown in Figure VII-5A and B where the regurgitant "v" wave of the wedge pressure disappeared. The diminution in mitral regurgitation may occur by three mechanisms:

1. If mitral regurgitation is due to papillary muscle dysfunction on the basis of myocardial ischemia, nitroglycerin causes a reduction in mitral regurgitation by improving myocardial perfusion and ischemia.[5,6]

2. By reducing the systemic arterial pressure;

3. By decreasing the heart size.

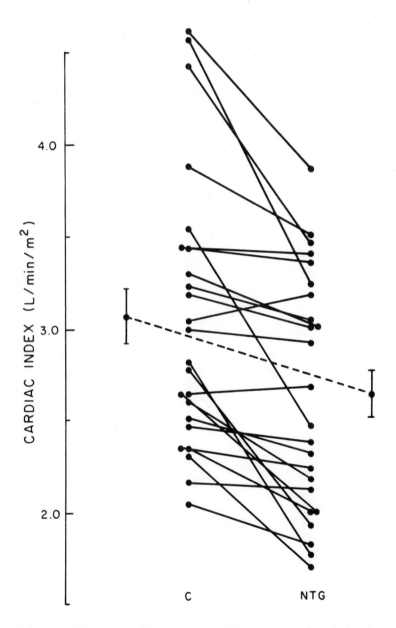

Fig. VII-2. A) Effect of sublingual nitroglycerin on cardiac index in patients ith normal-sized heart. C: Control NTG: Nitroglycerin.

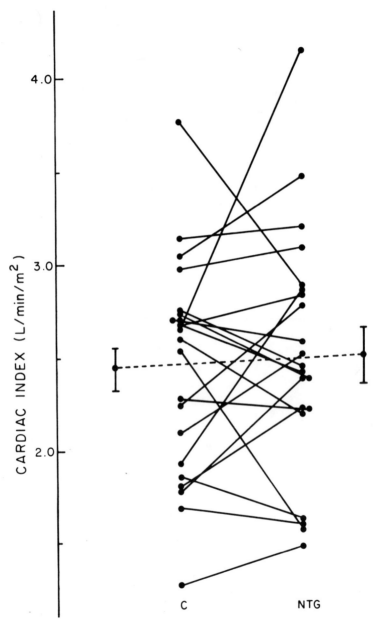

Fig. VII-2. B) Effect of nitroglycerin on cardiac index in patients with cardiomegaly.

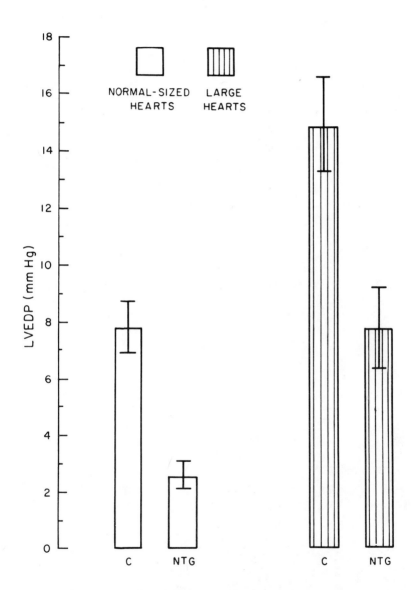

Fig. VII-3. Effect of sublingual nitroglycerin on left ventricular end-diastolic ressure in patients with normal-sized heart and patients with cardiomegaly.

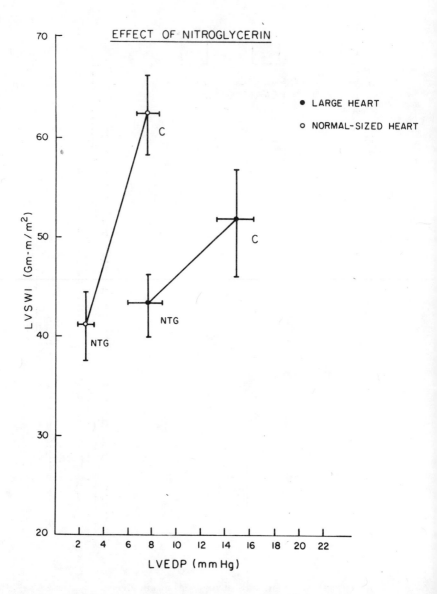

Fig. VII-4.   Left ventricular function curve relating left ventricular end-diastolic pressure to left ventricular stroke work index.

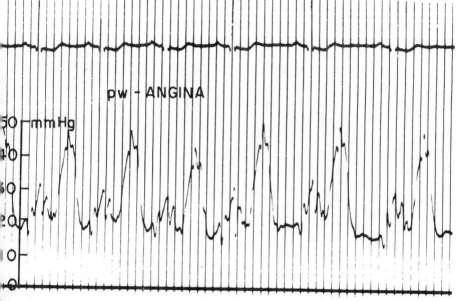

pw – ANGINA

mmHg

Fig. VII-5A. Effect of nitroglycerin on mitral regurgitation: A) Pulmonary wedge pressure showing a prominent regurgitant "V" wave during spontaneous angina.

Fig. VII-5B. After sublingual administration of 0.4 mg nitroglycerin, there is diminution in the pulmonary wedge pressure and the regurgitant "V" wave.

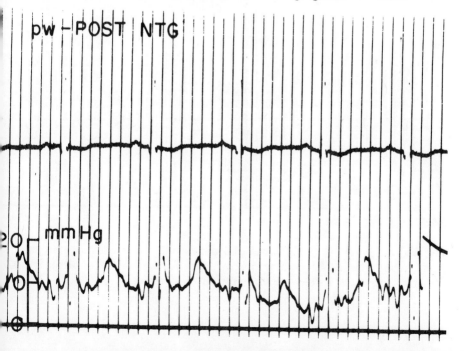

pw – POST NTG

mmHg

Thus the murmur of mitral regurgitation will become quiet or may actually disappear.

Currently there are three specific uses for the administration of sublingual nitroglycerin in cardiac catheterization:

1. As a hemodynamic intervention in idiopathic hypertrophic subaortic stenosis. Because of diminution in heart size, the degree of the outflow tract obstruction and thus the intraventricular systolic pressure gradient increases (Fig. VII-6).

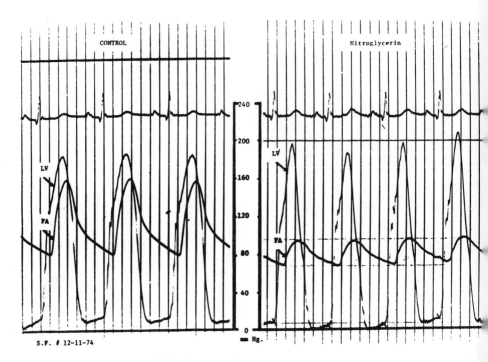

Fig. VII-6. Effect of nitroglycerin in a patient with idiopathic hypertrophic sub aortic stenosis. Due to diminution in heart size, the outflow tract obstruction is in tensified and thus the systolic pressure gradient is increased.

2. Prior to left ventriculography, to detect the areas of the heart which have reversible asynergy of contraction[7-10] (Fig. VII-7A and B). Since areas of hypokinesia or akinesia may be due to the underlying myocardial ischemia, they may be reversible after bypass surgery. In our laboratory, left ventriculograms are often performed 1–3 minutes after sublingual administration of 0.4 mg–0.8 mg nitroglycerin when there is diminution in the systolic pressure or an increase in the heart rate. Indeed if the "degree" of the improvement of contraction in the various zones of the heart is sought, a control left ventriculogram should be obtained before administration of nitroglycerin. The second left ventriculogram (post NTG) is then obtained in 20–30 minutes when the hemodynamic effect of contrast material is eliminated. Since coronary artery disease often affects different segments of the heart, the degree of asynergy is often analyzed in six different zones of the heart (Fig. VII-7A and B). Thus the longitudinal axis of the heart is divided into four equal parts by three chords (axes). The percent of shortening in each hemiaxis is then measured as the difference in length between systole and diastole and divided by the length in diastole.

3. To determine the therapeutic effects of unloading of the heart, especially in patients with cardiomegaly or cardiomyopathy in whom medical management primarily includes vasodilator therapy (see hemodynamic effects of nitroglycerin).

Amyl Nitrite[1]

Hemodynamic effects: The hemodynamic effects of amyl nitrite are primarily on the arteriolar side of the vascular system. Its rapid introduction into the circulation causes an abrupt and significant degree of arteriolar dilatation with a marked diminution in blood pressure which in turn causes a sympathetic

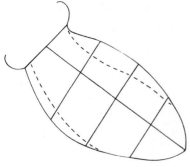

Fig. VII-7A. Schematic representation of left ventriculogram in right anterior oblique view. A) In control left ventriculogram, there is akinesia in the apical region.

A - CONTROL

Fig. VII-7B. When the left ventriculogram is repeated after sublingual nitroglycerin administration, the apical region contracts. Thus the diminished contraction in this area is most likely due to ischemia and not due to fibrosis or scar tissue.

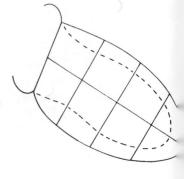

B - NTG

response by baroreceptor stimulation. Hence reflex venous constriction occurs which increases the venous return and cardiac output. The overall effect of amyl nitrite is thus a marked reduction in the arterial blood pressure, systemic vascular resistance, tachycardia and an increase in venous return and cardiac output. Its effect on the systemic circulation is more intense than on pulmonary circulation. Amyl nitrite is not generally used in the cardiac catheterization laboratory. It is, however, commonly used in conjunction with phonocardiography and echocardiography. Its value lies mainly in the detection of the following conditions:

1. *Idiopathic hypertrophic subaortic stenosis (IHSS):* Because of a reduction in the systemic arterial pressure, the murmur of IHSS becomes louder since the outflow tract obstruction is intensified. It should be mentioned that the systolic murmur of valvular aortic stenosis also becomes louder with amyl nitrite because of an increase in cardiac output.

2. *Mitral regurgitation:* After amyl nitrite inhalation, the mid-late systolic murmur of prolapsing mitral leaflet syndrome starts earlier in systole or may become pansystolic, and the systolic click will appear earlier. The murmur of rheumatic mitral regurgitation becomes quiet because of diminished systemic pressure.

3. *Mitral stenosis murmur vs. Austin Flint murmur:* Because of a diminution in the systemic vascular resistance, the degree of aortic regurgitation is decreased and therefore the early blowing diastolic murmur of aortic regurgitation becomes quiet. The diastolic rumble of mitral stenosis, on the other hand, increases in intensity with amyl nitrite because of an increase in cardiac output as well as tachycardia, both of which increase the left atrial pressure. The

Austin Flint murmur, however, diminishes with amyl nitrite since the degree of aortic regurgitation is decreased.

Isoproterenol

Isoproterenol infusion is used mainly as an intravenous provocative test for IHSS. Because of increased myocardial contractility, the degree of outflow tract obstruction is increased. In our cardiac catheterization laboratory, isoproterenol is administered by intravenous infusion of a solution of 1 μg/ml of isoproterenol (1 ampule of 0.2 mg isoproterenol is diluted in 200 ml of NSS or 5% DW). It is then administered by a micro-drip infusion set at a slow rate with gradual increase until a satisfactory chronotrophic effect is reached, or there is a significant increase in the intraventricular systolic pressure gradient. In addition, in patients with mitral stenosis, isoproterenol infusion causes an increase in the diastolic mitral valve gradient because of tachycardia and increased cardiac output (Fig. III-5, Chapter III).

Phenylephrine, Methoxamine and Angiotensin

These medications increase the systemic arterial pressure and act as a pressure load on the heart. They are not commonly used in routine catheterization studies.

Ergonovine Maleate Test for Coronary Arterial Spasm[11]

The ergonovine maleate test is used to detect coronary arterial spasm as the cause of Prinzmetal angina or its variant form. Ergonovine maleate is a weak vasoconstrictor which exerts its effect on the vascular musculature.

Technique of ergonovine testing: In our laboratory in patients suspected of having Prinzmetal angina, control left ventriculography and coronary cineangiography are performed without administration of nitroglycerin or any nitrite derivative. A temporary electrode pacemaker is inserted into the right heart as a precautionary measure since arrhythmias or heart block may occur often during Prinzmetal angina. After completion of the control angiographic studies, ergonovine maleate, 0.05 mg, is administered intravenously. Electrocardiograms and systemic arterial pressure are continuously monitored. If no angina or electrocardiographic changes are observed, ergonovine maleate is injected at dose levels of 0.1, 0.15, and 0.2 mg, at 5–10 minute intervals. If angina occurs at any time, coronary cineangiograms and, if possible, left ventriculograms are repeated and sublingual nitroglycerin or nitroglycerin solution (0.4 mg/ml) is administered intravenously or into the aortic root, after which the angiograms are repeated. Coronary cineangiograms should also be repeated after the 0.2 mg dose of ergonovine is administered without occurrence of angina or electrocardiographic abnormalities.

Figure VII-8 shows the schematic reproduction of coronary cineangiograms in a 40-year-old woman with Prinzmetal angina. The angiogram during control state, prior to the administration of nitroglycerin (A), did not reveal any obstructive disease. After administration of ergonovine (B), there was a marked reduction in the caliber of the left main coronary artery and its anterior descending branch with subtotal occlusion of the proximal circumflex and marginal branches and total occlusion of the circumflex branch in its distal part. The above changes disappeared after nitroglycerin administration (C). Similarly, the right coronary cineangiograms, which were normal during control state (A), showed a marked reduction in its caliber throughout its course (B) which reversed after nitroglycerin administration (C).

Figure VII-9 shows the electrocardiographic findings during the control state, ergonovine and nitroglycerin administration. Electrocardiographic leads II and V_5 were monitored throughout the procedure. During the control state, there was only slight ST

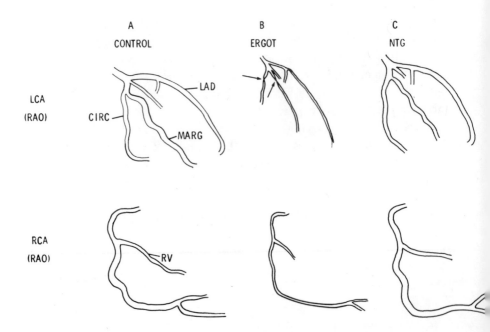

Fig. VII-8. Drawings from the cineangiographic frames in a patient with Prin
metal angina. A) Control coronary cineangiograms (without nitroglycerin). B) Core
nary cineangiograms after ergonovine administration; arrows show the occlusion
C) Coronary cineangiograms after nitroglycerin administration (see text).

depression in the above mentioned leads. The first electrocardiographic findings were "T" wave peaking which occurred prior to
angina (C). The patient subsequently developed angina and
bradycardia (D) with significant ST depression in lead V_5. There
were subsequent marked ST elevations which are best shown in
leads II and V_5 in F and G. Short runs of ventricular tachycardia occurred at the peak of angina, for which the patient was
treated with 50 mg of Lidocaine intravenously. After intravenous
and intra-aortic administration of nitroglycerin, the angina

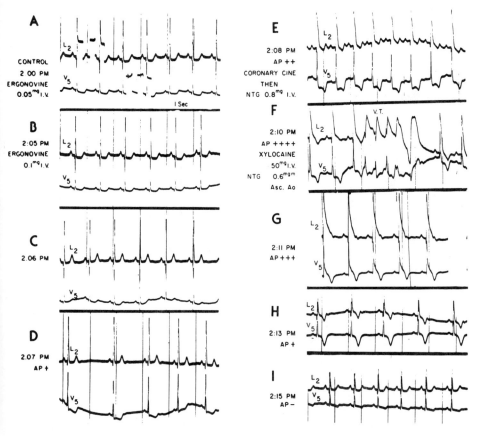

AP = ANGINA PECTORIS, NTG = NITROGLYCERINE, Asc. Ao = ASCENDING AORTA, VT = VENTRICULAR TACHYCARDIA

Fig. VII-9.   Electrocardiographic tracings, leads II and V_5 during ergonovine provocative test. A) Control tracing, after which ergonovine maleate 0.05 mg I. V. was administered. Since there were no electrocardiographic changes after five minutes, a dose of 0.1 mg I. V. was administered (B). The earliest electrocardiographic findings which were "T" wave peaking (C) occurred prior to angina. With the onset of angina, there was ST depression in lead V_5 and sinus bradycardia (D). At this time the patient developed systemic hypertension. Subsequently angina increased in intensity with further ST depression in V_5 and also in lead II (E). Nitroglycerin 0.8 mg was then administered intravenously. However, the angina became worse and the patient developed short runs of ventricular tachycardia. There was ST elevation in lead II (F). Lidocaine 50 mg was administered as intravenous bolus and nitroglycerin 0.6 mg was administered into the ascending aorta. The angina subsided in approximately one minute although there was now marked ST elevation (G). There was subsequent "T" wave inversion but no ST elevation (H) and the tracing was subsequently similar to the control tracing (I).

gradually subsided and the electrocardiogram returned to the control with no angina (I).

Ergonovine provocative testing should be done by experienced physicians since the coronary cineangiograms have to be repeated rapidly during the angina and electrocardiographic abnormalities. We prefer Sones technique over Judkins' for this test because the angiograms are performed rapidly with the same catheter. As was mentioned previously, a temporary pacemaker catheter should be positioned in the right heart for treatment of heart block if necessary. In case of severe hypertension, the patient may have to be treated with nitroprusside in addition to the intravenous nitroglycerin.

References

1. Mason, D. T., Zelis, R. and Amsterdam, E. A. Actions of the nitrites on the peripheral circulation and myocardial oxygen consumption: Significance in the relief of angina pectoris. Chest 59:296, 1971.
2. Campion, B. C., Frye, R. L. and Zitnik, R. S. Effects of nitroglycerin on capacitance vessels: A mechanism for reduction of left ventricular end-diastolic pressure. Mayo Clin. Proc. 45:573, 1970.
3. Williams, J. F., Jr., Glick, G. and Braunwald, E. Studies on cardiac dimensions in intact unanesthetized man. V. Effects of nitroglycerin. Circulation 32:767, 1965.
4. Hoeschen, R. F., Bousvaros, G. A., Klassen, G. A., Fam, W. M. and McGregor, M. Haemodynamic effects of angina pectoris, and of nitroglycerin in normal and anginal subjects. Brit. Heart J. 28:221, 1966.
5. Fam, W. M. and McGregor, M. Effect of coronary vasodilator drugs on retrograde flow in areas of chronic myocardial ischemia. Circ. Res. 15:355, 1964.
6. Fam, W. M., Nakhjavan, F. K., Sekely, P. and McGregor, M. The effects of oxygen breathing, nitroglycerin and dipyridamole on oxygen tension in healthy and ischemic areas of the myocardium. Proc. Int. Symp. Cardiovasc. Respir. Effects Hypoxia. Basel/New York, Karger, 1966, p. 375.

7. Helfant, R. H., Pine, R., Meister, S. G., Feldman, M. S., Trout, R. G. and Banka, V. S. Nitroglycerin to unmask reversible asynergy: Correlation with post coronary bypass ventriculography. Circulation 50:108, 1974.
8. Sniderman, A. D., Herscovitch, P., Marpole, D. and Fallen, E. L. Restoration of regional wall motion by nitroglycerin therapy in patients with left ventricular asynergy. Chest 66:5: 545, 1974.
9. Salel, A. F., Berman, D. S., DeNardo, G. L. and Mason, D. T. Radionuclide assessment of nitroglycerin influence on abnormal left ventricular segmental contraction in patients with coronary heart disease. Circulation 53:975, 1976.
10. Dumesnil, J. G., Ritman, E. L., Davis, G. D., Gau, G. T., Rutherford, B. D. and Frye, R. L. Regional left ventricular wall dynamics before and after sublingual administration of nitroglycerin. Am. J. Cardiol. 36:419, 1975.
11. Heupler, F. A., Jr., Proudfit, W. L., Razavi, M., Shirey, E. K., Greenstreet, R. and Sheldon, W. C. Ergonovine maleate provocative test for coronary arterial spasm. Am. J. Cardiol. 41: 631, 1978.

Appendix

Normal Values
Intracardiac Pressures

		Range (mmHg)
Right atrium	Mean	1 − 4
Right ventricle	Systolic	17 − 30
	Diastolic	1 − 4
Pulmonary artery	Systolic	17 − 30
	Diastolic	6 − 12
	Mean	9 − 19
Pulmonary wedge	Mean	5 − 13
Aortic	Systolic	90 − 140
	Diastolic	60 − 90
	Mean	70 − 100
Left ventricle	Systolic	90 − 140
	Diastolic	5 − 13
Left atrium	Mean	5 − 13

Oxygen consumption	143 ± 14.3 cm^3/m^2
Systemic arteriovenous O_2 diff.	4.1 ± 0.6 vol. %
Cardiac index	3.5 ± 0.7 L/min/m^2
Stroke index	46 ± 8.1 ml/beat/m^2
Systemic arterial O_2 saturation	96 − 100%

Resistances (*Dynes sec.cm^{-5}*)

Total peripheral resistance	1130 ± 178
Total pulmonary vascular resistance	205 ± 51
Pulmonary arteriolar resistance	67 ± 23

Left Ventriculographic Data

End diastolic volume index	50 − 95 ml/M^2
End systolic volume index	14 − 36 ml/M^2
Stroke volume	30 − 60 ml/m^2
Ejection fraction	0.56 − 0.78
Left ventricular mass	76 − 108 gm/m^2
Left ventricular wall thickness	7 − 12 mm
Mean velocity of circumferential fiber shortening	1.06 − 3.02 circ/sec

Electrophysiological Measurement		*Range* (*msec.*)
P-A interval:	Intra-atrial conduction time	25 − 45
A-H interval:	Atrioventricular nodal conduction time	60 − 125
H-V interval:	His-Purkinje conduction time	30 − 55
SRT:	Sinus recovery time	1150 − 1400
CSRT:	Corrected sinus recovery time	100 − 525
SACT:	Sinoatrial conduction time	28.5 − 153*

* varies significantly according to different investigators

INDEX

Page numbers in italics *indicate figures; "t" indicates tabular matter.*